Calorie
counting

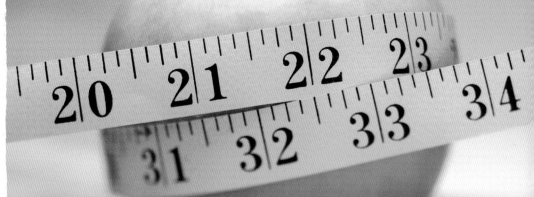

igloobooks

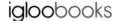

Published in 2014
by Igloo Books Ltd
Cottage Farm
Sywell
NN6 0BJ
www.igloobooks.com

Food photography and recipe development: Photocuisine UK
Front cover and additional images supplied courtesy of Thinkstock, Getty Images

Designed by Alyssa Peacock
Written by Alison Marlow

FIR003 0314
2 4 6 8 10 9 7 5 3
ISBN 978-1-78197-092-8

Printed and manufactured in China

Calorie
counting

Contents

Introduction 6

Get Motivated! 14

Goal Setting 16

Breakfast 18

Lunch 30

Main Meals 42

Snacks 60

Exercise 74

Week 1 80

Week 2 83

Week 3 86

Week 4 89

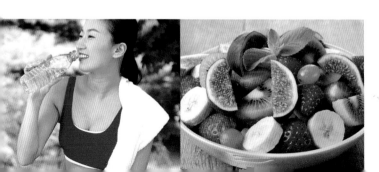

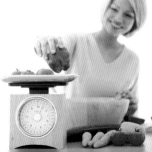

Stage 1 Success! 92

Week 5 94

Week 6 97

Week 7 100

Week 8 103

Stage 2 Success! 106

Week 9 108

Week 10 111

Week 11 114

Week 12 117

Stage 3 Success! 120

Calories List 122

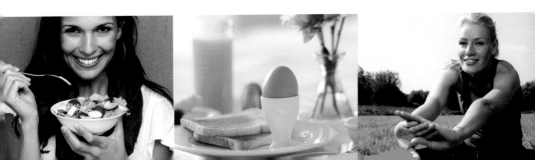

Success starts here!

Whether you want to lose a little or a lot of weight then this book is here to help. We've put together a 12-week weight loss plan that gives you lots of choice and masses of flexibility to help ensure that you don't get bored and give up on the way.

This little book is packed with plenty of ideas and advice to help you shed any excess pounds. And if you follow the guidelines and don't slip back into your old ways, you're sure to keep them off too.

Take it steady

Diets that promise fast weight loss are no good for you long term. You might drop the weight but the inevitable toughness of such regimes means that there's a good chance you'll pile it all back on again in no time. Likewise, steer clear of any diets that tell you to exclude food groups or rely on meal replacements.

Research shows that a steady weight loss programme works best. If you lose weight gradually, your body adjusts and you

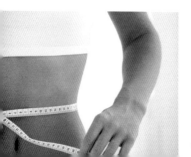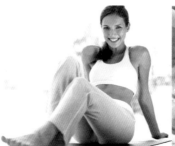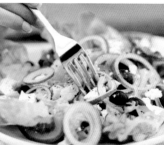

are more likely to keep the weight off.

For every pound you want to lose, you need to burn off 3,500 calories. So if you cut down your average daily intake by 500 calories a day, you'll lose a pound every seven days. With our diet you can expect to lose 1-2 lbs a week. Often you'll lose slightly more in the first week as your body adjusts and you lose excess water.

The Guideline Daily Amount (GDA) for women is 2000 calories a day.

This diet is based on 1500 calories a day. There is plenty for you to choose from to make sure you never get bored!

Each day you'll choose a:

- 250 calorie breakfast

- 300 calorie lunch

- 500 calorie dinner

- 150-calorie milk allowance – half a pint of semi-skimmed milk or 1 pint skimmed milk.

- 300 calorie snack

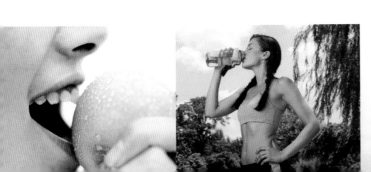
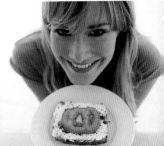

Drinks

Drink as much water as you like. Remember that water is essential to keep your body happy and healthy. Drink it plain, iced, or with a slice of fresh lemon or lime. You can also drink herbal teas, low-calorie fruit squashes, diet drinks, tea and coffee. Remember to use milk from your allowance if you like your tea and coffee white.

Calories – the lowdown

A calorie is a measurement of available energy. When food is metabolised it produces energy and that is measured in kilocalories (kCal). We call them calories for short.

Get the balance right

No single food contains all the nutrients your body needs. To ensure you not only lose weight but stay healthy, make sure you choose foods from all the food groups, protein, carbohydrate and fat. Ensure you have enough fibre too.

Protein

Proteins are the building blocks of the human body and are needed for growth and repair.

Good sources of protein include chicken and lean red meats, milk, eggs, fish and cheese.

Carbohydrate

Carbohydrates are our main source of energy. They are found in grains, pulses, fruits and vegetables.

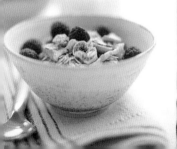
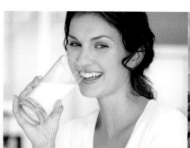
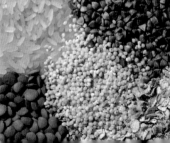

Fat

Everyone thinks of fat as a real baddie but some fat is needed in everyone's diet. Not all fats are the same and it's wise to steer clear of things containing saturated fats in favour of products with unsaturated fat.

Good fats include monounsaturates such as olive and rapeseed oils; omega-3 polyunsaturates, including oily fish and omega-6 polyunsaturates including sunflower and corn oil.

Fibre

Dietary fibre is a form of carbohydrate. It helps move food through the digestive system. Foods high in fibre add to a feeling of fullness and can help prevent you caving in and diving into the biscuit tin!

Always check with your doctor or medical practitioner before starting a diet, especially if you have any pre-existing medical condition or take medication. Taking exercise makes losing weight easier too: so always tell your doctor what kind of exercise you plan to do to ensure they feel this is suitable for you.

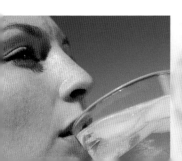
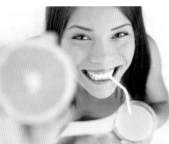
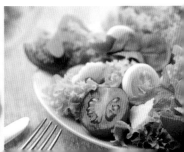

Don't be too hard on yourself…

Getting yourself into the 'diet zone' can feel quite liberating. Yes, you've actually decided to do something about those extra pounds. You've made a great commitment to your own health and wellbeing. That's brilliant in itself.

So if you have a hiccup along the way, don't take it to heart. Like any life-changing action, going on a calorie-controlled diet can take some getting used to. Along your weight-loss journey, some weeks will feel better than others. There will be days when your choice of dishes hits the spot perfectly, times when you just can't wait to leap out of the door and take that brisk walk.

But there might be other times when you feel things aren't going quite right, when you might even wonder if this diet is for you. These are the times when you need to be extra nice to yourself – look at how well you're doing and major on the positives.

Having a positive attitude towards your weight-loss effort can go a long way to succeeding long-term.

Think ahead

If you know you have events coming up that revolve around food, try and plan ahead. If there's a birthday celebration on the cards, or a wedding or party, then allow for that by ensuring you eat super-healthily a couple of days before.

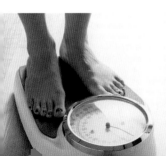 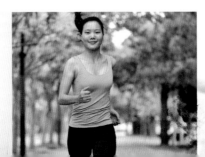 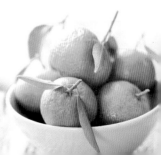

Weekend waywardness

Everyone likes to let their hair down a bit at the weekend, but don't let it ruin the hard work of the weekdays! Try and stick to the plan for most of your weekend meals, perhaps choosing one extra snack to celebrate your non-working days. When you get on those scales at the end of the week, you'll be so glad you didn't give in to the urge to splurge!

Ditch the guilt

If you do have a glitch, then ditch any feelings of guilt. We're all human! Feeling bad about slipping off the plan can sabotage success – if you let it. Consign any little food wobbles to the bin, and head for success by getting back on track.

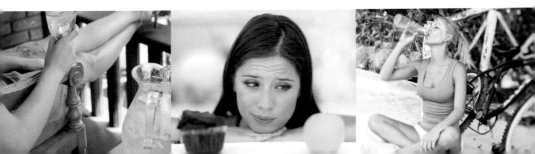

Find your own cheerleaders

Choosing to diet is a very personal decision – and one that some of the people around you might not always like. That's why it's important for you to rely on friends and family who really want you to succeed.

Having your own personal cheerleaders can work wonders for your morale and for watching the weight drop off. You know how encouraging it can be to have others tell you how well you're doing. Make sure you have someone like this to call on when things are going brilliantly – and even more importantly, on the days when it seems a little harder to stay on track.

We all have friends who seemingly try to stick the spanner into the spokes of our diets. You know, the sort that tries to encourage you to have that cream cake, or tries to talk you out of that swim you had planned. Be as firm as you can with them, as you're the one who will win out in the end!

Understand yourself

We don't have to be hungry to eat – that's why we all end up with a few unwanted pounds. There are so many reasons to eat, not least the fact that food of all kinds is absolutely yummy. Our emotions are behind our reasons for eating more often than we'd care to admit. But that needn't scupper your weight loss

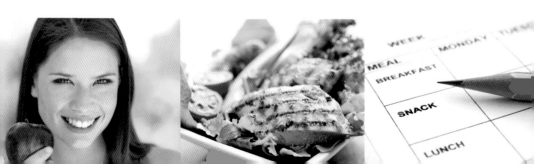

plans, so long as you know what type of eater you are.

Are you the kind to dip in the biscuit tin when you're a bit down, or downright bored? Maybe you love to celebrate good news with a curry or a cake, or perhaps you can't resist the spread of a family buffet or girls' night out?

Whether you're a comfort eater or a social eater, someone who picks without thinking or nibbles when bored – this diet plan can work well for you. Sit down for a few minutes and work out what kind of eater you are. Then you can help plan your days to avoid the times and situations when you might be tempted to revert to your old habits.

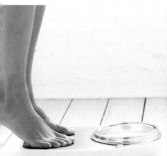
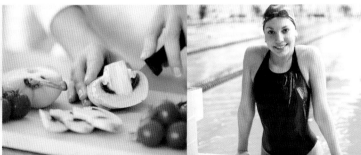

Get Motivated!

You're already determined to do this – that's why you're reading this book! But here are a few more ideas to help you keep that motivation, and momentum, going in the right direction over the whole 12 dieting weeks.

Psyche yourself up

Visualise the new you. Picture yourself in those clothes that haven't fitted comfortably in months. Imagine your new look in the mirror. See and feel how you're going to be a few weeks down the line.

Picture this

Have a photograph of yourself at your heaviest, and one of you as you'd like to be. It could be a shot of you in slimmer days or a celebrity whose body you most admire. If you want to keep the photos from prying eyes, stick them on to the inside of a cupboard door in the kitchen – that way you'll have the perfect reminder to stay on track.

Health benefits

Being overweight isn't great news for our health, so dropping even just a few pounds can

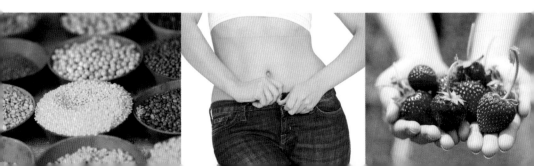

make a difference. Losing weight can help reduce raised blood pressure and cut down the risk of heart disease. It can also reduce strain on your joints. As you lose weight, you become more mobile, making it easier to fit exercise into a regular routine. And even better, it can boost your mood and improve self-esteem.

Tester outfits

It could be a dress you want to slim into, or a pair of jeans that are that bit too tight. Your tester clothes are all about you and what you want. At the end of every week (or each four-week stage, if you prefer), get out your tester clothes and see how close you're getting to slipping back into them. Don't try them on unless you want to, just hold the clothes against you and see how far you've come. You'll be dancing round the room wearing those favourites in no time!

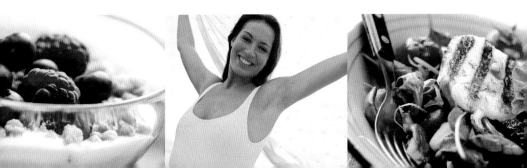

Goal Setting

Before you start...
...have a goal in mind.

Research shows that if you have something definite to aim for, then you're more likely to stay on track.

It could be a celebration on the horizon, a wedding, a holiday or simply a desire to get back into that sexy bra and brief set that fitted like a glove last year. Choose a goal personal to you, because you're doing this for you. No-one else, just you.

You've got to want to do this for yourself. It's no good telling yourself you'll lose weight for your boyfriend or kids. If you do that, chances are you won't make it to the finish line.

Be selfish for once! Make this all about you. Yes, you! You're going to be brilliant at it. And a few weeks down the line, you'll be so glad you opened this little diet book.

Goals

Setting realistic goals is essential. You build success on success. Start small and then you're more likely to stick to the simple changes you make. That way,

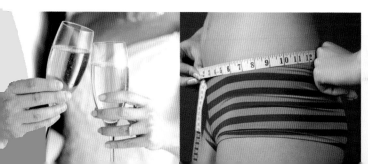
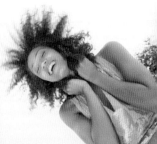

you'll get the results you want.

And don't be too hard on yourself. If you make things too tough or try to achieve too much, you'll get disheartened and may end up piling the pounds back on again.

Think short-term. This diet plan runs for 12-weeks but set yourself a weekly goal as well as a four-weekly goal. By doing that, it means you're taking baby steps on the road to a new you.

If you think in seven-day chunks, it helps you stay focused and the little changes you make along the way make a big difference in the long run.

Step on the scales once a week, no more! Your weight fluctuates throughout the day so always weigh yourself at the same time in the same clothes each time.

Record your weight in the space provided.

Also, take your measurements at the beginning of Week One and every four weeks. Sometimes when weight loss seems a little slow, you'll find you're still losing vital inches!

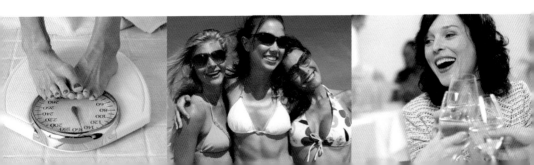

Breakfast

A good breakfast will set you up for the day, leave you feeling positive and full of determination to stick to the plan. As we all know, every day is different – some mornings you'll be dashing to get out of the house on time, others you'll have a nice gentle start.

That's why we've included a huge range of breakfast options, from things you can eat on the go, to tasty savouries you can take your time over. Ring the changes by chopping and changing – research shows that boredom with the same old choices is one of the things that can lead to you losing interest in a weight-loss plan.

Use your breakfast choice to boost your mood. Feeling fruity? There are many lovely choices including fresh and

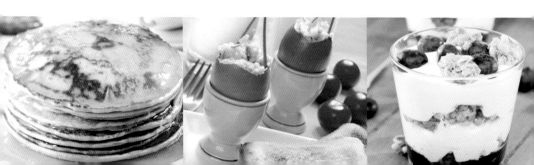

juicy fruits. Can't get going without something crunchy? Then take a look at our toast and cereal options. Remember, if you want to get your morning off to a refreshingly good start, squeeze half a lemon into a glass of cool water and sip it slowly. It can pep up your tastebuds as well as doing the crucial trick of rehydrating you after a long night's sleep.

Don't usually eat breakfast? Who says you have to eat breakfast the moment you wake up? If you're the sort that needs a coffee to get you going, then do what works for you and have your breakfast a little later on in the morning. Whatever you do, don't skip this vital meal altogether.

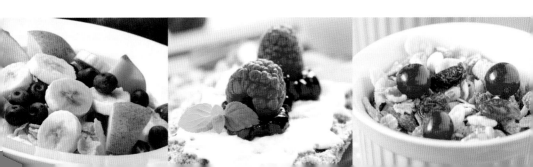

Breakfast

Don't be tempted to skip breakfast. It kick starts your metabolism for the day and also prevents the temptation to snack on high-calorie foods mid-morning. Even if you're in a rush, take five minutes to eat breakfast. We've devised a range of meal ideas for days when you're dashing and times when you can be a little more leisurely.

People who are most successful at losing weight – and keeping it off – opt for breakfast every single day. Choose from any of the ideas in this section. They're all light, nutritious and will make every day worth getting up for!

Scrambled Eggs with Ham

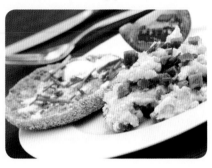

Serves 4
250 calories per serving
Prep time: **5 minutes**
Cooking time: **3 minutes**

6 large eggs, 75 g lean ham, cubed
60 ml low-fat plain yoghurt
2 wholemeal rolls, halved
a small bunch of chives, chopped

Break the eggs carefully into a small saucepan and beat them lightly with a fork. Stir in the ham.

Put the pan over a medium heat and stir constantly until the eggs scramble to your liking.

Stir in half the yoghurt and spoon onto hot plates. Spread the rolls with the remaining yoghurt and serve with the eggs. Sprinkle with chives.

Granary French Toast

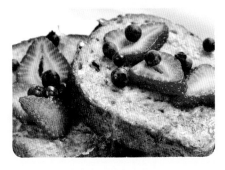

Serves 4
250 calories per serving
Prep time: 5 minutes
Cooking time: 8 minutes

1 large egg, 100 ml skimmed milk
4 thick slices wholemeal granary bread
5 sprays low-calorie spray oil
3 tbsp honey, 4 strawberries, sliced
a small handful of blueberries

Beat the egg with the milk and
brush it over both sides of the
bread. Spray a large frying pan with
oil and heat until it starts to sizzle.

Fry the bread for 2 minutes on
each side or until golden brown.
Brush the toast with honey and
serve with the sliced strawberries
and blueberries scattered over.

Simple Scrambled Eggs

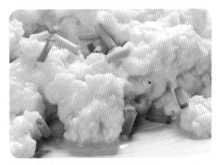

Serves 2
185 calories per serving
Prep time: 2 minutes
Cooking time: 3 minutes

4 large eggs
a small bunch of chives, chopped

Break the eggs into a small
saucepan and beat them
lightly with a fork.

Put the pan over a medium
heat and stir constantly until the
eggs scramble to your liking.

Spoon onto warm plates
and sprinkle with chives.

Breakfast Fruit Salad

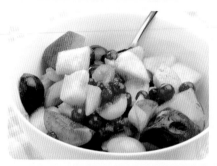

Serves 4
130 calories per serving
Prep time: 10 minutes

200 g plums, stoned
200 g nectarines, stoned
200 g pear, cored
200 g apple, cored
150 g seedless grapes, halved
100 g blackberries
100 g redcurrants
4 tbsp unsweetened grape juice

Cut the plums, nectarines, pear and apple into bite-sized pieces.

Mix with the grapes, blackberries and redcurrants and spoon over the grape juice.

Blackberry & Apple Smoothie

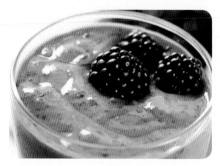

Serves 2
180 calories per serving
Prep time: 2 minutes

200 g blackberries
300 ml apple juice
300 ml low-fat plain yoghurt

Reserve 6 blackberries and put the rest in a blender with the apple juice and yoghurt.

Blend for 2 minutes or until smooth then pour into glasses and top with the reserved blackberries.

Scrambled Egg Cups

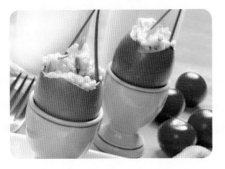

Serves 2
190 calories per serving
Prep time: 8 minutes
Cooking time: 3 minutes

2 slices of white bread, 2 eggs, chives, chopped, 4 cherry tomatoes

Toast the bread under a hot grill and keep warm. Break the eggs carefully into a small saucepan and reserve the larger half of each shell. Beat the eggs lightly with a fork.

Put the pan over a medium heat and stir constantly until the eggs scramble to your liking. Spoon the eggs back into the reserved shells and sprinkle with chives.

Serve with warm toast and cherry tomatoes.

Strawberry & Banana Skewers

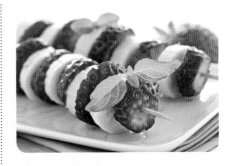

Serves 2
220 calories per serving
Prep time: 5 minutes

240 g banana, sliced
200 g strawberries, sliced
60 ml runny honey
4 sprigs of mint

Thread the fruit onto 4 skewers, alternating between banana and strawberry slices.

Drizzle over the honey and garnish with mint sprigs.

Raspberry Crispbread

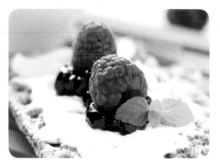

Serves 1
84 calories per serving
Prep time: 2 minutes

1 rye crispbread
1 tbsp low fat soft cheese
2 tsp raspberry jam (jelly)
2 raspberries
mint leaves to garnish

Spread the crispbread with low fat soft cheese and top with the jam and raspberries.

Garnish with mint leaves.

Redcurrant Muesli

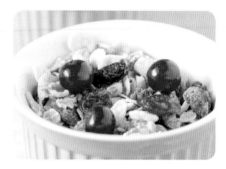

Serves 4
132 calories per serving
Prep time: 5 minutes

50 g jumbo porridge oats
20 g toasted wheat flakes
20 g millet flakes
50 g sultanas
150 g redcurrants

Mix the oats with the wheat flakes, millet flakes and sultanas and store in an airtight jar until ready to use.

Stir in the redcurrants just before serving.

Fruity Cereal

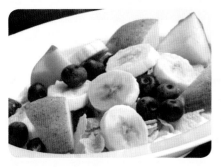

Serves 1
268 calories per serving
Prep time: 5 minutes

30 g cornflakes
100 ml skimmed milk
½ banana, sliced
½ ripe pear, cored and cubed
50 g blueberries

Measure the cornflakes into
a bowl and pour over the milk.

Top with the fruit and
serve straight away.

Fruit and Flakes

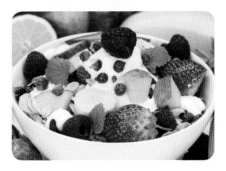

Serves 4
188 calories per serving
Prep time: 5 minutes

15 g cornflakes, 25 g jumbo porridge
oats, 20 g toasted wheat flakes,
40 g dried cranberries, 200 g 0% fat
Greek yoghurt, 50 g redcurrants,
125 g raspberries, 150 g strawberries,
halved, 1 ripe peach, stoned and
chopped, 1 banana, sliced, mint
leaves to garnish

Mix the cornflakes with
the oats, wheat flakes and
dried cranberries and store in
an airtight jar until ready to use.

Divide the muesli mixture between
four bowls and top with the
yoghurt. Top with the fresh fruit and
garnish with mint leaves.

Berry Breakfast Pots

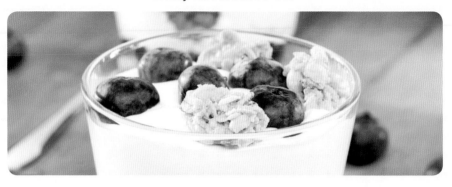

Serves 2
204 calories per serving
Prep time: **10 minutes**
Cooking time: **4 minutes**

100 g blueberries, 1 tbsp caster (superfine)
sugar, 200 g 0% fat Greek yoghurt, 50 g granola

Reserve a few blueberries for decoration
and put the rest in a saucepan with the
sugar and a tablespoon of water. Cover
the pan and simmer over a low heat for
4 minutes or until the blueberries start to
burst and soften. Leave to cool.

Divide the blueberry mixture between two
glasses and top with half the yoghurt.
Sprinkle over half of the granola, then
spoon in the rest of the yoghurt.

Top with the remaining granola and
the reserved blueberries.

Syrup Pancakes

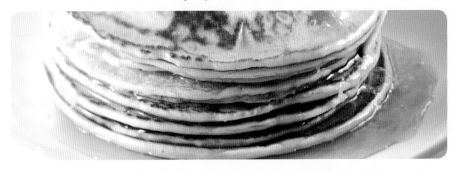

Serves 4
256 calories per serving
Prep time: **5 minutes**
Cooking time: **20 minutes**

125 g plain (all purpose) flour, 1 tsp baking powder, 150 ml skimmed
milk, 1 large egg, beaten, 1 tbsp butter, 100 ml maple syrup

Mix the flour and baking powder in a bowl then pour
in the milk and egg and use a whisk to gradually
incorporate all of the flour from around the outside.

Melt the butter in a frying pan then whisk it into the batter.
Put the buttered frying pan back over a low heat.

Spoon a small amount of the batter into the pan and cook for
2 minutes or until small bubbles start to appear on the surface.
Turn the pancake over with a spatula and cook the other
side until golden brown and cooked through.

Repeat until all the batter has been used, keeping
the finished batches warm in a low oven, then pour
over the syrup before serving.

Summer Fruit Yoghurt

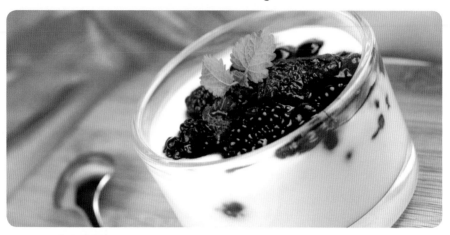

Serves 2
114 calories per serving
Prep time: **10 minutes**
Cooking time: **5 minutes**

100 g frozen summer fruit
1 tbsp caster (superfine) sugar
200 g 0% fat Greek yoghurt

Put the fruit in a saucepan
with the sugar and a tablespoon
of water. Put on the lid and simmer
gently for 5 minutes or until the
fruit starts to burst and soften.
Leave to cool completely.

Divide the yoghurt between
two glass bowls and spoon
the compote on top.

Branflakes with Strawberries & Yoghurt

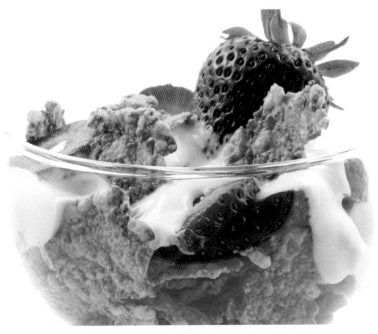

Serves 1
210 calories per serving
Prep time: **2 minutes**

45 g branflakes
60 g strawberries, sliced
100 ml low-fat plain yoghurt

Mix the branflakes and sliced
strawberries together in a bowl
and spoon over the yoghurt.

Lunch

While breakfast gives you a vital energy boost first thing, a light but tasty and filling lunch can help fuel your afternoons. Eating a good lunch also helps you keep away from the office vending machine, the biscuit tin at home and the vast array of naughties that face every dieter who's out and about these days.

Our lunches have something for every midday muncher – from hot and warming comfort foods for cooler days, to colourfully crispy salads. There is plenty for those of you who have to pack a lunch to take with you, along with leisurely choices for when you have more time to cook and relax. On the days when you're not running around, make an event of lunch. Take time out to sit down at a table and savour every mouthful. To ensure you stay hydrated,

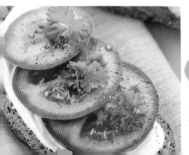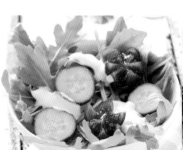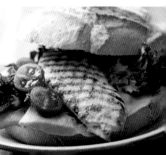

accompany your lunch with a tall cool glass of water or other low-calorie drink.

Don't be tempted to skip lunch as doing this can lead to a huge drop in energy mid to late afternoon, at a time that your resolve might be feeling weak. You don't want to sabotage your excellent progress by finding yourself jumping for a sugary chocolate bar to give you an artificial boost. Many of the recipes can easily be doubled or tripled if you're catering for others as well as yourself.

There are plenty of ideas for every kind of luscious lunch, from that old reliable standby, the humble jacket potato to the more exotic. Make your lunches as colourful as possible, with the addition of very low calorie salad vegetables – peppers, leafy salads, tantalising tomatoes and cute slices of cucumber.

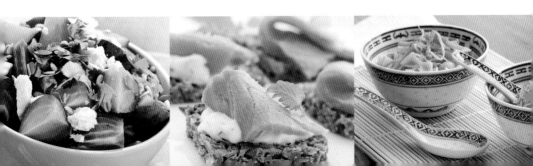

Lunch

Baked Potato with Blue Cheese

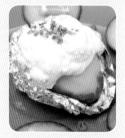

Serves 1

300 calories
per serving

Prep time:
10 minutes

Cooking time:
1 hour

1 large baking potato
15 g blue cheese
55 g low-fat cottage cheese
1 tbsp chives, chopped

Preheat the oven to 200ºC
(180º fan) 400F, gas 6.

Wrap the potato in foil and
bake in the oven for 1 hour.

Put the blue cheese and cottage
cheese in a blender and blend
until smooth.

When the potato is ready,
carefully unwrap the foil, spoon
the dressing on top and
sprinkle with chives.

Garden Vegetable Omelette

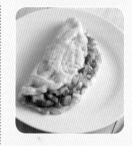

Serves 1

230 calories
per serving

Prep time:
5 minutes

Cooking time:
5 minutes

10 sprays of low-calorie spray oil,
½ onion, chopped, ½ courgette,
chopped, 1 large tomato, chopped,
2 large eggs, beaten

Add 5 sprays of oil to a large
frying pan and fry the onion for
2 minutes. Add the courgette
and tomato and season well with
salt and pepper.

Heat another 5 sprays of oil in
a non-stick frying pan and add
the eggs. Cook until they start to
set around the edge then use a
wooden spatula to draw the sides
in, letting the gaps fill up with
uncooked egg.

Repeat until the top is set to
your liking then spoon the
vegetable filling into the centre,
fold over and serve.

Tuna Pasta Salad

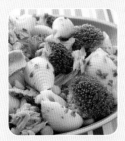

Serves 4

300 calories
per serving

Prep time:
10 minutes

Cooking time:
12 minutes

225 g dried pasta shells, 150 g broccoli florets, 200 g canned tuna, 2 tsp lemon juice, 150 g canned sweetcorn, 1 tbsp flat leaf parsley, chopped

Bring 2 large pans of salted water to the boil. Cook the pasta in one pan for 12 minutes or until al dente. Drain and plunge into cold water to cool. Drain again. Meanwhile, cook the broccoli in the second pan for 4 minutes or until just tender. Reserve 1 tbsp of the cooking water then drain and plunge into cold water to cool. Drain again.

Drain the tuna, reserving 2 tsp of the brine, and break it into large flakes. Mix the reserved brine with the lemon juice and dilute to taste with the broccoli cooking water. Toss the cooled pasta and broccoli with the tuna, sweetcorn and dressing. Sprinkle with parsley.

Smoked Salmon Frittata

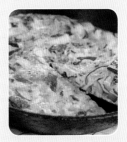

Serves 6

120 calories
per serving

Prep time:
5 minutes

Cooking time:
15 minutes

10 sprays of low-calorie spray oil, 2 shallots, finely chopped, 1 large courgette, chopped, 6 large eggs, 100g smoked salmon, chopped

Preheat the grill. Add 5 sprays of oil to a pan and fry the shallots for 2 minutes. Add the courgette, season well and cook for 5 minutes.

Beat the eggs and stir in the salmon. Scrape the courgette mix into the eggs then return the pan to the heat.

Add another 5 sprays of oil to the pan. Stir the eggs to incorporate the courgettes then pour into the pan.

Cook over a low heat until the frittata has set round the edges, but is still runny in the centre.

Put the pan under the grill to finish cooking the top then leave to cool a little before serving.

Leek and Shiitake Soup

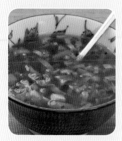

Serves 4

150 calories
per serving

Prep time:
5 minutes

Cooking time:
15 minutes

6 dried shitake mushrooms, 2 tbsp
sunflower oil, 2 leeks, trimmed and
sliced, 1 clove of garlic, crushed,
2 cm fresh root ginger, finely grated,
4 tbsp rice wine, 1 litre beef stock,
150 g fresh shiitake mushrooms,
sliced, 2 tbsp soy sauce, 1 tsp
arrowroot powder

Put the dried mushrooms in a
bowl and pour over boiling water
to cover. Heat the oil and fry the
leeks for 5 minutes. Add the garlic
and ginger and cook for 2 minutes,
then add the wine and simmer.

Add the stock and bring to
the boil. Strain the soaked
mushroom's liquor and add
to the pan. Slice the soaked
mushrooms and add them to the
pan with the fresh mushrooms.

Boil for 2 minutes then add the
soy sauce and season. Mix the
arrowroot with 1 tbsp cold water
then add it to the soup.

Rocket with Yoghurt Dressing

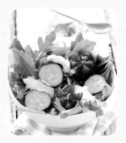

Serves 2

60 calories
per serving

Prep time:
5 minutes

2 tbsp low-fat plain yoghurt
2 tbsp low-fat mayonnaise
1 tbsp lemon juice
2 medium tomatoes
80 g cucumber, sliced
80 g rocket

Mix together the yoghurt,
mayonnaise and lemon juice with a
pinch of salt to make the dressing.

Slide a sharp paring knife into the
side of one tomato on the
diagonal, then take it out, turn
the knife 90º and slide it in again
next to the first cut. Repeat all the
way around the tomato to make
a zigzag pattern then carefully twist
the 2 halves apart. Repeat with
the second tomato.

Fill 2 bowls with the rocket
and arrange the cucumber and
tomatoes on top, then spoon
over the dressing.

Mushroom Pancake Omelette

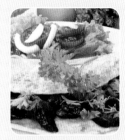

Serves 1

200 calories
per serving

Prep time:
2 minutes

Cooking time:
10 minutes

10 g butter, 125 g chestnut mushrooms, sliced, 1 large egg, 2 tbsp flat leaf parsley, chopped

Melt the butter in a large frying pan and use a pastry brush to brush a small non-stick frying pan with a thin layer of melted butter. Set aside.

Fry the mushrooms in the rest of the melted butter for 8 minutes or until any liquid has evaporated and they turn golden brown.

Heat the second buttered frying pan. Gently beat the egg then add it to the pan and swirl it around to cover the bottom in a thin even layer. Reduce the heat so that the egg cooks through slowly to make a pancake-thin omelette.

Season the mushrooms and stir in the chopped parsley then spoon into the centre of the omelette and serve.

Grilled Chicken Salad

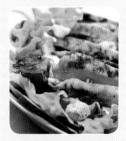

Serves 2

290 calories
per serving

Prep time:
5 minutes

Cooking time:
8 minutes

2 x 150 g skinless chicken breasts, 1 tsp olive oil, ½ tsp herbs de Provence, ½ clove of garlic, crushed, 60 ml low-fat plain yoghurt, 15 ml lemon juice, 2 large tomatoes, quartered, 80 g cucumber, sliced, 80 g lettuce, 20 g croutons

Preheat the grill. Brush the chicken breasts with olive oil, sprinkle with the dried herbs and season well with salt and pepper.

Grill for 4 minutes on each side or until cooked through and golden brown.

Mix the garlic, yoghurt and lemon juice to make the dressing and season to taste with salt and pepper. Mix together the tomato, cucumber and lettuce and drizzle with dressing.

Slice the chicken and lay it on top of the salad then sprinkle with croutons.

Vegetable Soup

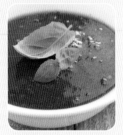

Serves 2

164 calories
per serving

Prep time:
10 minutes

Cooking time:
15 minutes

1 tbsp olive oil, a pinch of chilli (chili) flakes, 3 cloves of garlic, crushed, 1 onion, quartered and sliced, ½ tsp smoked paprika, 1 tbsp concentrated tomato puree, 400 g canned tomatoes, chopped, 100 g frozen mixed vegetables, defrosted, 800 ml vegetable stock, a small bunch of basil leaves

Heat the olive oil in a saucepan, then fry the chilli, garlic and onion over a medium heat for 5 minutes.

Stir in the paprika and tomato puree and cook for 1 minute, then stir in the tomatoes and vegetables. Pour in the stock then simmer for 5 minutes.

Transfer the soup to a liquidiser. Reserve a few basil leaves for garnish, then add the rest to the soup and blend until smooth. Season to taste with salt and pepper, then pour into two warm bowls and garnish with basil.

Pasta Shell Soup

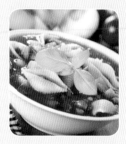

Serves 2

276 calories
per serving

Prep time:
2 minutes

Cooking time:
20 minutes

2 tsp olive oil, 1 onion, quartered and sliced, 3 cloves of garlic, crushed, ½ tsp smoked paprika, 1 tbsp concentrated tomato puree, 400 g canned tomatoes, chopped, 800 ml vegetable stock, 100 g frozen mixed vegetables, 75 g pasta shells, a few sprigs of basil to garnish

Heat the olive oil in a saucepan, then fry the onion over a medium heat for 5 minutes or until translucent.

Add the garlic and fry for 2 more minutes, then stir in the paprika and tomato puree.

Add the chopped tomatoes and stock to the pan. When it starts to simmer, add the frozen vegetables.

When it starts to simmer again, add the pasta and cook for 10 minutes or until al dente.

Ladle into two warm bowls and garnish with basil.

Beetroot with Feta

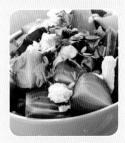

Serves 2

277 calories
per serving

Prep time:
30 minutes

Cooking time:
1 hour

350 g whole unpeeled candy stripe beetroot, 350 g whole unpeeled golden beetroot, 2 tbsp cider vinegar, 1 tsp runny honey, 50 g Feta cheese, 2 tbsp sunflower seeds, 2 tbsp flat leaf parsley, roughly chopped

Preheat the oven to 190°C (170° fan) / 375F / gas 5. Wrap each beetroot in a sheet of foil, then bake until tender all the way through (30 minutes for small beetroots and up to an hour for big ones).

Leave until cool enough to handle, then unwrap and slip off the skins. Cut the beetroots into bite-sized chunks and divide between two bowls.

Stir the vinegar into the honey with a pinch of salt and drizzle over the beetroot. Crumble over the Feta and sprinkle with sunflower seeds and parsley before serving.

Pasta Stir-Fry

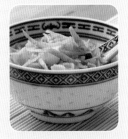

Serves 4

161 calories
per serving

Prep time:
2 minutes

Cooking time:
8 minutes

75 g pasta shells, 2 tbsp sunflower oil, 1 tbsp root ginger, finely chopped, 2 cloves of garlic, finely chopped, 2 medium carrots, peeled and julienned, ¼ Chinese cabbage, shredded, 100 g beansprouts, 2 tbsp rice wine, 2 tbsp light soy sauce

Cook the pasta in boiling salted water according to the packet instructions or until al dente. Drain well.

Heat the oil in a wok and stir-fry the ginger and garlic for 30 seconds. Add the carrots and cabbage and stir-fry for 2 minutes, then add the beansprouts and pasta and cook for 1 more minute.

Pour in the rice wine and soy sauce, then cover with a lid and steam for 2 minutes.

Divide between 4 warm bowls and serve immediately.

Tomato Spaghetti

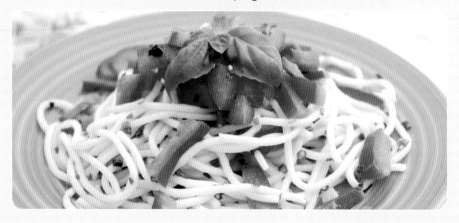

Serves 1
285 calories per serving
Prep time: 2 minutes
Cooking time: 12 minutes

75 g spaghetti
100 g ripe tomatoes, chopped
1 tbsp basil leaves, chopped,
plus extra to garnish
1 tbsp fresh chives, chopped

Cook the spaghetti in boiling salted
water until al dente, according to the
packet instructions.

Drain it well, then toss with the tomato
and its juices and the fresh herbs.

Transfer to a warm plate and garnish
with basil.

Grilled Chicken Roll

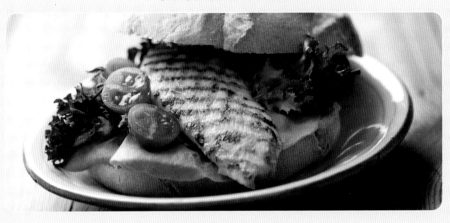

Serves 1
314 calories per serving
Prep time: **5 minutes**
Cooking time: **12 minutes**

1 x 125 g skinless chicken breast
1 white crusty roll
2 lettuce leaves
2 cherry tomatoes, halved

Heat a griddle pan until smoking hot.
Season the chicken breast liberally all
over with salt and pepper.

Griddle the chicken for 12 minutes,
turning every 3 minutes, or until it's
cooked through and nicely marked.

Cut the roll in half and fill with the
lettuce, tomatoes and chicken. Eat
immediately.

Pumpernickel Bites

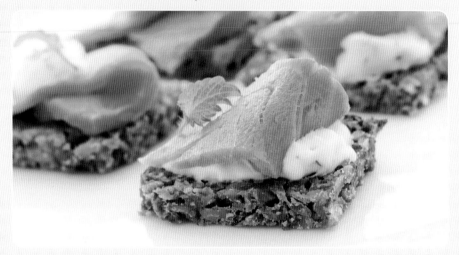

Serves 1
144 calories per serving
Prep time: 5 minutes

1 tbsp low fat soft cheese
1 tsp lemon balm leaves, chopped,
plus extra to garnish
1 slice pumpernickel bread
1 slice smoked salmon, quartered

Mix the cheese with the chopped lemon
balm and spread it over the bread.

Cut the bread into four pieces
and top each one with a quarter
of a slice of smoked salmon.

Garnish with extra lemon balm.

Tomato on Rye

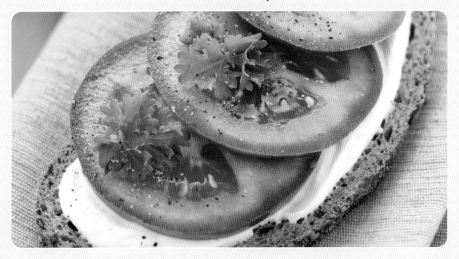

Serves 1
134 calories per serving
Prep time: 2 minutes

1 thin slice rye bread
2 tbsp low fat soft cheese
½ medium tomato, sliced
curly parsley to garnish

Spread the bread with
the cheese and arrange the
tomato slices on top.

Garnish with parsley
and sprinkle with freshly
ground black pepper.

Main Meals

The main meal of the day will leave you feeling well-nourished and satisfied, and guard against any temptation to raid the cupboards in search of midnight fare. Our recipes are easy to make and give fabulous results. Enjoy the whole process of meal creation, from chopping the vegetables to serving out on to fine crockery.

They say we eat first with our eyes and while you're on this meal plan, really take the time to make your food choices works of art, rather than refuelling. If you've taken time over the meal then you're more likely to really appreciate every mouthful.

Keep an eye on the number of servings in each recipe and make sure you divide all servings equally to ensure you take in the correct number of calories. There's everything here, from deliciously rustic

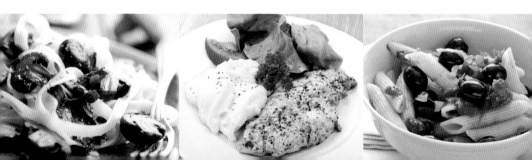

meals, to vegetarian options and delicate dishes that beg to be eaten slowly so you can savour every mouthful.

Don't forget to really taste your food and chew every mouthful. People who eat slowly and really let their tastebuds get to work can often have more success than scoffers who bolt their food and finish in no time. When it comes to eating aim to be more tortoise than hare – nice and slowly does it!

Mix and match the recipes over the 12 weeks. You're sure to have a few firm favourites but try to be adventurous too – now's the time to try foods you'd never considered before. Remember: a lot of weight loss successes come from you getting to know yourself so much better. Decide on your main meal choice at least a day before so you can ensure you have all the right ingredients to hand.

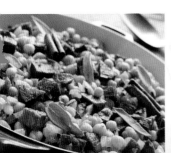
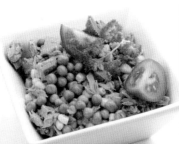
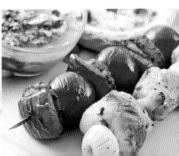

Main meals

Steak Fajitas

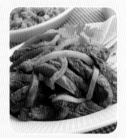

Serves 4

490 calories
per serving

Prep time:
5 minutes

Cooking time:
6 minutes

30 ml sunflower oil
500 g lean rump steak, sliced
1 red pepper, sliced
1 yellow pepper, sliced
1 green pepper, sliced
35 g fajita seasoning mix
8 soft flour tortillas

Heat the oil in a frying pan
and stir-fry the steak for
4 minutes or until cooked through.

Add the peppers and seasoning
mix and stir-fry for 2 minutes.

Spoon onto a warm plate and
serve with the tortillas.

Mediterranean Chicken Skewers

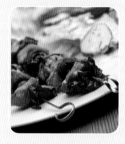

Serves 2

500 calories
per serving

Prep time:
5 minutes

Cooking time:
6 minutes

250 g chicken breast pieces
120 g sundried tomatoes in oil, drained
300 g button mushrooms

Preheat the grill.

Thread the chicken onto
4 skewers, alternating with the
sundried tomato pieces and
whole mushrooms.

Brush the skewers with a little of
the oil from the tomato jar and grill
for 6 minutes or until cooked
through, turning occasionally.

Chilli Con Carne Soup

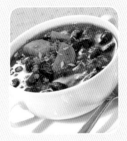

Serves 4

370 calories
per serving

Prep time:
2 minutes

Cooking time:
30 minutes

2 tbsp olive oil
2 shallots, finely chopped, 1 red chilli,
finely chopped, 2 cloves of garlic,
crushed, 1 tbsp fresh thyme leaves,
½ tsp Cayenne pepper, 400 g lean
beef mince, 500 g tomato passata,
500 ml beef stock, 3 large carrots,
thickly sliced, 400 g canned kidney
beans, drained

Heat the oil in a large saucepan
and fry the shallot and chilli for
3 minutes, stirring occasionally.

Add the garlic, thyme and Cayenne
pepper and cook for 2 minutes,
then add the beef mince.

Fry the mince until it starts
to brown then add the passata,
stock and carrots and simmer
for 20 minutes.

Stir in the kidney beans and cook
for 5 more minutes, then ladle
into warm bowls to serve.

Griddled Pork with Curried Rice

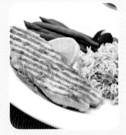

Serves 2

320 calories
per serving

Prep time:
30 minutes

Cooking time:
20 minutes

100 g basmati rice, 2 tsp mild curry
powder, 2 x 120 g lean pork leg
steaks, 4 sprays of low-calorie spray
oil, 100 g French beans, trimmed

Soak the rice in cold water for
30 minutes then rinse. Put the rice
in a saucepan with 320 ml of cold
water and stir in the curry powder.

Heat the pan until it starts to boil,
then put the lid on and turn the
heat down. Cook the rice for
10 minutes then turn off the heat
and leave for 5 minutes.

Cook the beans in boiling salted
water for 4 minutes then drain.
Meanwhile, heat a pan until
smoking hot. Spray the steaks
with oil and season.

Griddle for 2 minutes on each side.
When the rice is ready, serve with
the pork and beans.

Piri Piri Turkey with Yoghurt Mash

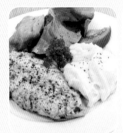

Serves 4

360 calories
per serving

Prep time:
2 hours

Cooking time:
25 minutes

1 tbsp piri piri seasoning mix
2 tbsp olive oil
1 tbsp lemon juice
4 x 100 g turkey breast steaks
800 g potatoes, peeled and chopped
100 ml low-fat plain yoghurt

Mix the piri piri seasoning with the olive oil and lemon juice and rub it into the turkey. Leave to marinate for 2 hours. Preheat the grill.

Boil the potatoes in salted water for 15 minutes or until tender then drain.

Meanwhile, cook the turkey steaks under the grill for 3 minutes on each side or until cooked through.

Mash the potatoes and stir in the yoghurt to make a fluffy consistency then taste for seasoning.

Serve on warm plates.

Salmon with Lemon and Almonds

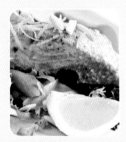

Serves 2

490 calories
per serving

Prep time:
5 minutes

Cooking time:
6 minutes

2 x 150 g salmon fillets
20 g blanched almonds
1 lemon
1 tsp honey
1 tsp Dijon mustard
3 tbsp extra virgin olive oil
60 g mixed salad leaves

Preheat the grill. Season the salmon with salt and pepper and cook for 6 minutes, turning halfway through.

Roughly chop the almonds and pare the lemon with a zester.

Mix together the honey and mustard and whisk in 2 tbsp of juice from the lemon. Whisk in the oil and taste for seasoning then stir in the almonds and lemon zest.

Arrange the salad leaves on 2 plates and top with the salmon. Spoon over the dressing and serve immediately.

Chilli No-Carne

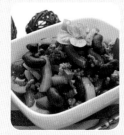

Serves 4

500 calories
per serving

Prep time:
2 minutes

Cooking time:
30 minutes

2 tbsp olive oil, 2 shallots, finely
chopped, 1 red chilli, finely chopped,
2 cloves of garlic, crushed, ½ tsp
Cayenne pepper, 400 g veggie mince,
1 red pepper, sliced, 1 yellow pepper,
sliced, 1 green pepper, sliced, 400 g
canned tomatoes, chopped, 500 ml
vegetable stock, 200 g brown rice,
400 g canned kidney beans, drained,
a few sprigs of fresh basil

Heat the oil in a large saucepan
and fry the shallots and chilli for
3 minutes. Add the garlic and
Cayenne pepper and cook for
2 minutes, then add the mince.

Fry the mince until brown then add
the peppers and stir-fry for 2 more
minutes. Add the tomatoes and
stock and simmer for 15 minutes.

Meanwhile, cook the rice according
to the packet instructions. Stir the
kidney beans into the chilli and
cook for 5 minutes, then garnish
with basil and serve with the rice.

Jewelled Rice

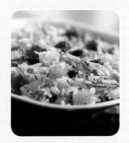

Serves 4

321 calories
per serving

Prep time:
30 minutes

Cooking time:
30 minutes

240 g basmati rice, 1 tbsp olive oil, 2
cloves of garlic, crushed, 2 slices Parma
ham, chopped, a pinch of saffron, 320
ml vegetable stock, 6 dried apricots,
chopped, 40 g dried cranberries, 2 tbsp
flat leaf parsley, chopped

Soak the rice with a pinch of
salt for 30 minutes, then rinse.

Heat the oil in a saucepan,
then fry the garlic and ham for
30 seconds. Add the drained
rice and stir-fry for 2 minutes.

Stir the saffron into the stock, then
pour it into the saucepan. When it
starts to boil, cover the pan, and
simmer gently for 15 minutes.

When the time is up, sprinkle
in the apricots and cranberries
then leave to stand off the heat
for 10 minutes.

Fluff up the rice grains with a
fork whilst stirring through the
parsley, then serve.

Spaghetti with Seafood Ragu

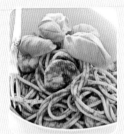

Serves 4

500 calories
per serving

Prep time:
2 minutes

Cooking time:
15 minutes

400 g dried spaghetti, 1 tbsp olive oil, 2 cloves of garlic, crushed, 1 red chilli, finely chopped, 300 ml tomato passata, 300 g raw king prawns, 200 g cooked crab meat, a few sprigs of basil

Cook the spaghetti in boiling salted water for 12 minutes or until al dente.

Meanwhile, heat the oil in a large frying pan and fry the garlic and chilli for a few seconds.

Pour in the passata and simmer for 5 minutes then stir in the prawns.

Cook for 2 minutes or until they have turned opaque then stir in the crab.

Season well with salt and pepper. Drain the spaghetti and stir it through the sauce. Serve in warm bowls, garnished with basil.

Turkey Mole

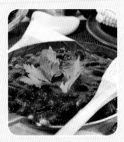

Serves 4

440 calories
per serving

Prep time:
5 minutes

Cooking time:
25 minutes

2 tbsp olive oil, 2 shallots, finely chopped, 1 red chilli, finely chopped, 2 cloves of garlic, crushed, 2 tsp smoked paprika, 300 g turkey breast, chopped, 200 ml vegetable stock, 300 g tomato passata, 240 g canned sweetcorn, drained, 400 g canned kidney beans, drained, 50 g dark chocolate, grated

Heat the oil in a large saucepan and fry the shallot and chilli for 3 minutes, stirring occasionally.

Add the garlic and smoked paprika and cook for 2 minutes, then add the turkey pieces.

Fry the turkey until it starts to brown then add the passata and stock and simmer for 15 minutes.

Stir in the sweetcorn and kidney beans and cook for 5 more minutes, then stir in the grated chocolate. Taste for seasoning before serving.

Spaghetti with Prawns

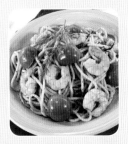

Serves 2

480 calories
per serving

Prep time:
2 minutes

Cooking time:
15 minutes

200 g dried spaghetti, 1 tbsp olive oil, 1 clove of garlic, crushed, 150 g raw king prawns, 100 g cherry tomatoes, halved, 2 tbsp fresh dill, chopped

Cook the spaghetti in boiling salted water for 12 minutes or until al dente.

Meanwhile, heat the oil in a large frying pan and fry the garlic for a few seconds. Using half of the tomatoes, squeeze them into the pan with your fingers and discard the skins.

Add the prawns and cook, stirring occasionally, until they turn pink. Stir in the dill and season well with salt and pepper. Add a few tablespoons of the pasta water to the sauce and stir to emulsify.

Drain the pasta and toss it with the sauce. Serve in warm bowls, garnished with the remaining tomato halves.

Pea and Parmesan Risotto

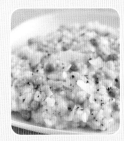

Serves 2

490 calories
per serving

Prep time:
5 minutes

Cooking time:
15 minutes

1 litre vegetable stock, 15 g butter, 1 onion, finely chopped, 1 clove of garlic, crushed, 150 g risotto rice, 20 g Parmesan, 200 g frozen peas, defrosted

Heat the stock in a saucepan. Melt half the butter in a pan and fry the onion for 5 minutes.

Add the garlic and cook for 2 minutes then stir in the rice. Add 2 ladles of stock. Cook, stirring occasionally, until most of the stock has been absorbed then add the next 2 ladles.

Continue in this way for 15 minutes until the rice is tender.

Finely grate half of the Parmesan and stir it through with the peas and the rest of the butter, then cover the pan and take off the heat to rest for 4 minutes. Serve warm, sprinkled with Parmesan.

Chicken Salad

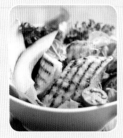

Serves 1

303 calories
per serving

Prep time:
5 minutes

Cooking time:
12 minutes

1 x 125 g skinless chicken breast,
4 lettuce leaves, ½ avocado, peeled
and stoned, 2 cherry tomatoes,
halved, 1 tbsp lemon juice,
a few basil leaves

Heat a griddle pan until
smoking hot and season the
chicken breast liberally all over
with salt and pepper.

Griddle the chicken for
12 minutes, turning every
3 minutes, or until it's cooked
through and nicely marked. Cut the
chicken across into 3 big pieces.

Arrange the lettuce leaves in
a bowl and top with the avocado,
tomatoes and chicken.

Sprinkle with lemon juice
and scatter over the basil
leaves before serving.

Turkey Stir-Fry

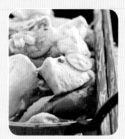

Serves 4

152 calories
per serving

Prep time:
2 minutes

Cooking time:
9 minutes

2 tbsp sunflower oil, 2.5 cm fresh root
ginger, thinly sliced, 2 cloves of garlic,
finely chopped, 1 red chilli (chili), finely
chopped, 1 green chilli (chili), thinly
sliced, 200 g turkey breast, cut into
chunks, 2 medium carrots, peeled
and julienned, 1 green pepper,
cut into chunks, 2 tbsp rice wine,
2 tbsp light soy sauce

Heat the oil in a wok and
stir-fry the ginger, garlic and
chillies for 30 seconds.

Add the turkey breast and
stir-fry for 3 minutes, then add
the vegetables and stir-fry for
a further 3 minutes.

Pour in the rice wine and
soy sauce, then cover with a lid
and steam for 2 minutes.

Divide between 4 warm bowls
and serve immediately.

Thai Prawn Curry

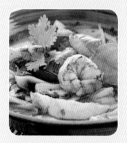

Serves 4

181 calories
per serving

Prep time:
2 minutes

Cooking time:
6 minutes

1 tsp sunflower oil, 2 tbsp red Thai curry paste, 400 ml vegetable or fish stock, 100 ml coconut milk, 2 kaffir lime leaves, 1 lemongrass stalk, bashed, 100 g button mushrooms, quartered, 150 g raw king prawns, peeled, 200 g tofu, sliced, 1 large red chilli (chili), sliced

Heat the oil in a wok and stir-fry the curry paste for 1 minute. Stir in the stock and coconut milk, then add the lime leaves and lemongrass to the pan.

When the curry starts to simmer, add the mushrooms, prawns, tofu and chilli. Simmer for 3 minutes or until the prawns turn opaque and curl up.

Ladle into four warm bowls and serve.

Grilled Salmon

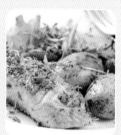

Serves 1

344 calories
per serving

Prep time:
5 minutes

Cooking time:
15 minutes

100 g new potatoes, 1 x 120 g salmon fillet, 1 tsp butter, 2 tsp lemon juice, 1 tbsp fresh thyme leaves, 20 g rocket (arugula), 2 cherry tomatoes, halved

Boil the potatoes in salted water for 15 minutes or until tender, then drain well.

Meanwhile, season the salmon with salt and pepper, then cook under a hot grill for 4 minutes on each side or until just cooked in the centre. Remove and discard the skin.

Toss the potatoes with the butter, lemon juice and half of the thyme, then transfer to a warm plate with the salmon.

Arrange the rocket and tomatoes on the side, then scatter over the rest of the thyme.

Chicken Skewers

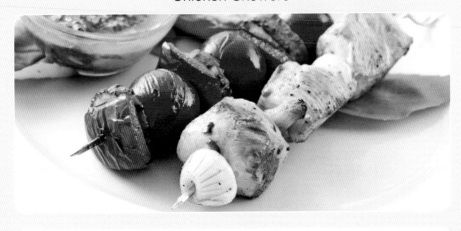

Serves 2
313 calories per serving
Prep time: 10 minutes
Cooking time: 10 minutes

1 x 125 g skinless chicken breast, ½ medium courgette (zucchini), 2 salad onions, ½ red pepper, 6 cherry tomatoes, 1 toasted bagel, halved, 2 tbsp pesto

Cut the chicken breast into 6 even-sized chunks and cut the courgette into 6 slices. Cut each salad onion into 3 pieces and cut the pepper into 6 pieces.

Thread the tomatoes, pepper and courgette onto two metal skewers and thread the chicken and salad onions onto two more.

Cook the skewers under a hot grill for 10 minutes or until the chicken is cooked through, turning regularly.

Serve one of each skewer per person with half a bagel and the pesto for dipping.

Chorizo and Chickpeas

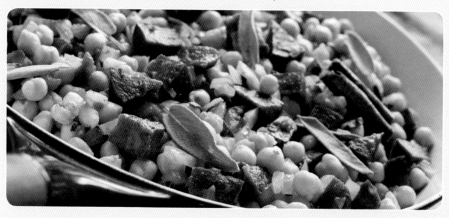

Serves 4
211 calories per serving
Prep time: **2 minutes**
Cooking time: **12 minutes**

100 g chorizo, cubed, 1 onion, finely chopped,
2 cloves of garlic, crushed, 1 cinnamon stick,
halved, 1 tbsp fresh sage leaves, chopped, plus
extra to garnish, 450 g canned chickpeas (garbanzo
beans), drained, 200 ml vegetable stock

Fry the chorizo in a hot frying pan for 2 minutes
to release some of the oil. Add the onion,
garlic, cinnamon and sage and cook over
a low heat for 5 minutes to soften.

Add the chickpeas and stock to the pan and
simmer for 5 minutes or until the stock has
almost all evaporated.

Garnish with sage leaves before serving.

Lime-Griddled Chicken

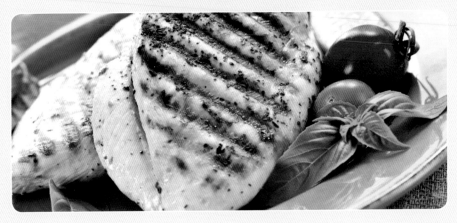

Serves 1
315 calories per serving
Prep time: **35 minutes**
Cooking time: **12 minutes**

1 lime
2 x 125 g skinless chicken breasts
2 cherry tomatoes
a few basil leaves

Finely grate the zest of the lime, then squeeze
the juice. Mix the zest and juice with a pinch of
salt and pepper, then pour it over the chicken
breasts and leave to marinate for 30 minutes.

Heat a griddle pan until smoking hot. Griddle
the chicken for 6 minutes on each side, or until
cooked through and nicely marked.

Serve the chicken with cherry tomatoes
and basil leaves to garnish.

Thai Beef Curry

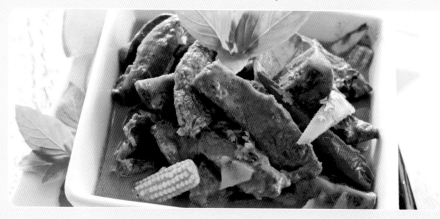

Serves 4
178 calories per serving
Prep time: **2 minutes**
Cooking time: **8 minutes**

1 tsp sunflower oil, 2 tbsp red Thai curry paste, 1 x 225 g sirloin steak, trimmed of fat, 12 baby corn cobs, 150 g canned bamboo shoots, drained, ½ aubergine (eggplant), cubed, 1 large red chilli (chili), 400 ml beef stock, 100 ml coconut milk, holy basil to garnish

Heat the oil in a wok and stir-fry the curry paste for 1 minute.

Thinly slice the steak and stir-fry it in the paste until browned. Add the baby corn, bamboo shoots, aubergine and chilli to the pan and turn to coat in the paste.

Stir in the stock and coconut milk then simmer for 3 minutes.

Ladle into four warm bowls and serve garnished with holy basil.

Olive Penne

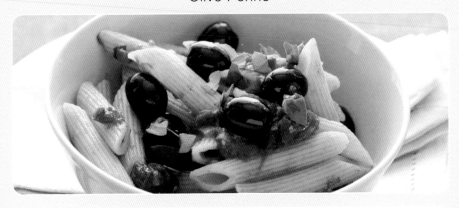

Serves 1
372 calories per serving
Prep time: 2 minutes
Cooking time: 12 minutes

75 g penne pasta, 1 tsp olive oil, 1 clove of garlic, crushed, a pinch of chilli (chili) flakes , 100 g ripe tomatoes, chopped, 10 black olives, pitted, 1 tbsp basil leaves, chopped

Cook the penne in boiling salted water until al dente, according to the packet instructions.

While the pasta is cooking, heat the oil in a small saucepan and fry the garlic and chilli for 30 seconds.

Add the chopped tomatoes and cook for 4 minutes, then stir in the olives.

Drain the pasta and stir it into the tomato pan, then tip it into a warm bowl and garnish with basil.

Asian Noodles

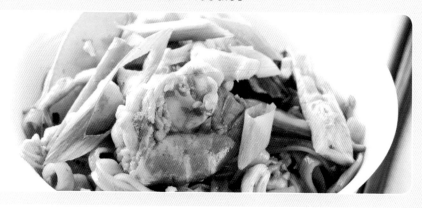

Serves 2
373 calories per serving
Prep time: 5 minutes
Cooking time: 8 minutes

125 g dried medium egg noodles, 2 tsp sunflower oil, 50 g skinless chicken breast, sliced, 100 g mangetout peas, 4 raw king prawns, peeled with tail left intact, 2 tbsp rice wine, 2 tbsp light soy sauce, 2 tbsp oyster sauce, 2 spring onions, sliced diagonally, 2 tbsp cashew nuts

Boil a saucepan of water, then submerge the noodles, turn off the heat and leave to soften for 5 minutes.

Meanwhile, heat the oil in a wok, then stir-fry the chicken for 2 minutes. Add the mangetout and prawns and stir-fry for 2 more minutes.

Stir in the rice wine, soy sauce and oyster sauce, then cover with a lid and steam for 2 minutes.

Stir in the drained noodles, spring onions and cashew nuts, then divide between 2 bowls and serve.

Tuna and Marrowfat Pea Salad

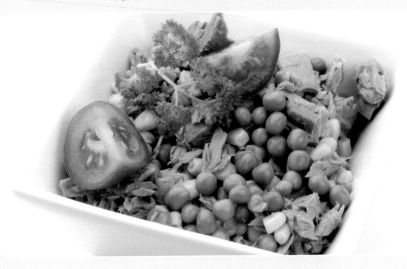

Serves 4
240 calories per serving
Prep time: 5 minutes

200 g canned tuna, 150 g canned sweetcorn,
300 g canned marrowfat peas, 2 tbsp extra
virgin olive oil, 1 tbsp lemon juice, 1 tsp honey,
2 medium tomatoes, quartered

Drain the tuna, sweetcorn and
peas and mix together.

Whisk together the oil, lemon juice and
honey and season with salt and pepper.

Toss the dressing with the tuna and
vegetables and spoon into bowls.

Top with the tomato wedges.

Mushroom Tagliatelle

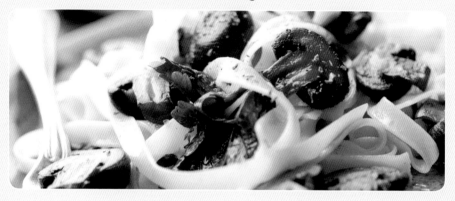

Serves 1
321 calories per serving
Prep time: **2 minutes**
Cooking time: **12 minutes**

75 g tagliatelle, 1 tsp butter, 1 clove of garlic, crushed,
100 g chestnut mushrooms, sliced,
2 tbsp flat leaf parsley leaves

Cook the tagliatelle in boiling salted water until al
dente, according to the packet instructions.

Meanwhile, heat the butter in a pan, then fry the
garlic for 30 seconds. Add the mushrooms and fry
for 2 minutes, then add 4 tbsp of the pasta cooking
water. Season with salt and pepper, stir in the parsley
leaves then simmer gently until the pasta is ready.

Drain the tagliatelle, then tip it into the mushroom
pan and turn to coat in the juices.

Transfer to a warm bowl and serve immediately.

Snacks

Snacks can make or break a diet. If you deprive yourself of treats you're more likely to hit the wall and head for the biscuit tin or the chocolate shop when you're feeling down. Many diets fail because people are too hard on themselves – they tend to 'ban' the little snacks that liven up their days. With our plan there's no need to quit snacking. We've devised a yummy, scrummy selection of snacks of 300 calories or less. If you factor in enough calories to allow for a little of what you fancy, you're more likely to stick to your plan and reach your ultimate goal.

There are savoury fillers and fruity choices, piquant treats and sweet, chewy choices for those times when you really need a mouthful of flavour. When you have a snack is entirely up to you – use them

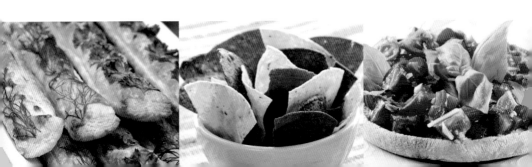

as a reward at the end of the day, or eat them in your old 'danger' times – when you're tempted to dunk a doughnut or crash out the bumper bag of crisps.

These snacks can be your diet-saving buddies – and even when your 12 weeks are up, we bet you'll still be choosing them over the old fatty choices! Make your snack time into an occasion –

sort out your snack, then sit down and savour it. Switch off the TV, turn off your phone and really relish your personal treat moment.

Before you start snacking though, try having a drink first, such as a glass of water or a cup of tea. Often we think we're hungry when really we're thirsty.

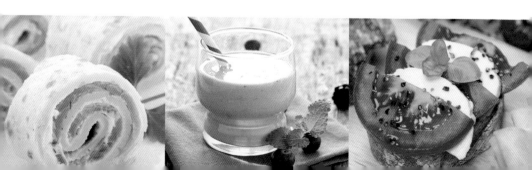

Snacks

Strawberry Meringues

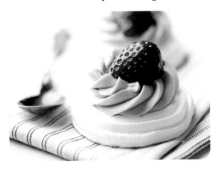

Serves 4
115 calories per serving
Prep time: 10 minutes

125 g low-fat cream cheese,
15 g icing sugar, 4 tbsp strawberry
syrup, 4 meringue nests, 4 large
strawberries

Beat the cheese with the
sugar and syrup until smooth
then spoon into a piping bag.
Pipe a swirl in the centre of each
nest and top with a strawberry.

Tomato and Basil Bruschetta

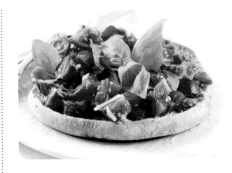

Serves 4
135 calories per serving
Prep time: 2 minutes

3 tomatoes, 1 shallot, chopped, basil,
torn, 2 tbsp extra virgin olive oil,
2 ciabatta rolls, halved

Chop the tomatoes and mix with
the shallot, basil and olive oil.
Season and spoon ¼ onto
each ciabatta half.

Hummus

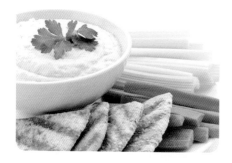

Serves 4
250 calories per serving
Prep time: 5 minutes

400 g tin of chickpeas, drained,
1 clove of garlic, crushed, 2 tbsp tahini
paste, 2 tbsp olive oil, 4 tbsp lemon
juice, 2 pita bread, 2 large carrots,
2 celery sticks

Put the chickpeas in a blender with
the garlic, tahini paste, olive oil, half
of the lemon juice and plenty of salt
and pepper. Blend until smooth.
Taste for seasoning and add extra
lemon juice or salt as required. To
make a thinner consistency, add
a few tablespoons of water and
blend again.

To serve, toast the pita breads
and cut them into wedges. Cut the
carrots and celery into batons.

Banana Milkshake

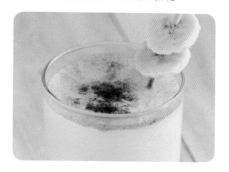

Serves 2
220 calories per serving
Prep time: 2 minutes

3 ripe bananas, sliced
350 ml skimmed milk
8 ice cubes
½ tsp ground cinnamon

Reserve 4 slices of banana
and thread onto 2 cocktail
sticks for a garnish.

Put the rest of the banana
into a blender with the milk
and ice cubes.

Blend for 2 minutes or until
smooth and thick.

Pour into 2 glasses and
sprinkle with cinnamon.

Banana and Honey Flapjacks

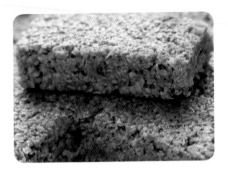

Makes 10
280 calories per serving
Prep time: 5 minutes
Cooking time: 30 minutes

2 ripe bananas, 100 ml honey,
100 g low-fat baking margarine,
500 g rolled porridge oats

Preheat the oven to 190ºC (170º fan) 375F, gas 5. Put the bananas in a blender with the honey and margarine and blend until smooth.

Stir the mixture into the oats then spoon into a greased baking tin and level the surface. Bake for 30 minutes or until golden brown and cooked through. Cut into squares while still warm but leave to cool completely before removing from the tin.

Crescent Moon Cookies

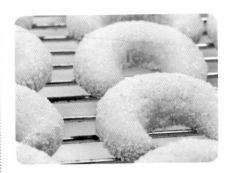

Makes 24
260 calories per serving (2 cookies)
Prep time: 2 hours 30 minutes
Cooking time: 20 minutes

225 g ground almonds, 275 g plain flour, 100 g icing sugar, 1 egg white, beaten, ½ tsp almond essence, 100 g low-fat margarine, 20 g caster sugar

Mix the almonds, flour and sugar in a bowl. Stir the egg white and almond essence into the margarine then mix with the dry ingredients, into a soft dough. Chill for 2 hours.

Preheat the oven to 170ºC (150º fan) 325F, gas 3. Shape into 24 moons and roll them in caster sugar.Place on 2 lined trays and bake for 20 minutes. Transfer to a wire rack to cool.

Sweet Pretzels

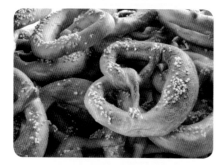

Makes 4
300 calories per serving
Prep time: 2 hours 30 minutes
Cooking time: 10 minutes

300 g bread flour, ½ tsp dried yeast,
15 g butter, melted, 1 tsp salt, 1 tbsp
egg white, beaten, sugar nibs,
210 ml warm water

Mix the flour, yeast, butter and
salt in a bowl and stir in the water.
Form into a dough and knead
for 10 minutes. Prove for 1 hour.
Divide into 4 and roll each into a
sausage. Twist into pretzel shape
and place on a baking tray. Prove
for 45 minutes.

Preheat oven to 220ºC (200º fan)
425F, gas 7. Brush them with egg-
white, sprinkle with sugar nibs and
bake for 10 minutes.

Quick Chips and Dip

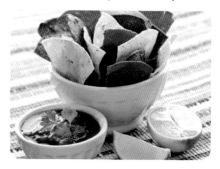

Serves 1
169 calories per serving
Prep time: 2 minutes

¼ lime, juiced
½ tsp smoked paprika
50 g tomato salsa
28 g tri-colour tortilla chips

Stir the lime juice and
paprika into the salsa,
then serve with the
tortilla chips.

Salmon Pinwheels

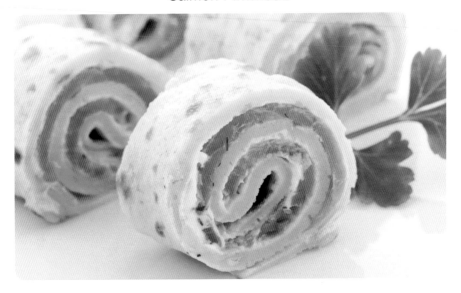

Serves 1
232 calories per serving
Prep time: 5 minutes

1 flour tortilla
1 tbsp low fat soft cheese
1 tsp dill, finely chopped
2 slices smoked salmon

Spread the tortilla with cheese
and sprinkle with dill.

Lay the salmon slices on top,
then roll up tightly and cut into
3 cm slices.

Basil Strawberries

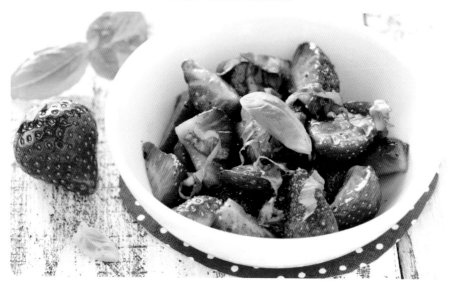

Serves 2
86 calories per serving
Prep time: 35 minutes

400 g strawberries
1 tbsp caster (superfine) sugar
1 tbsp basil leaves, shredded

Cut the strawberries into quarters,
then sprinkle with sugar and a
good grind of black pepper.

Leave to macerate for
30 minutes, then scatter over
the basil and serve.

Madeline Fingers

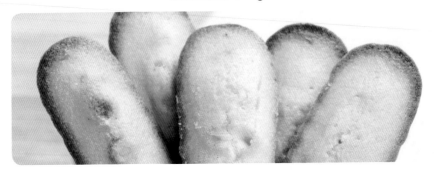

Makes 12
152 calories per serving
Prep time: **1 hour 30 minutes**
Cooking time: **12 minutes**

110 g butter, 55 g plain (all-purpose) flour, 55 g ground
almonds, 110 g icing (confectioners') sugar, 3 large egg whites

Heat the butter until it foams and smells nutty,
then leave to cool. Combine the flour, almonds and
sugar in a bowl and whisk in the eggs whites. Pour the
cooled butter through a sieve into the bowl and whisk
it into the mixture. Leave the cake mixture to rest in the
fridge for an hour.

Preheat the oven to 160°C (140° fan) / 325F / gas 3
and oil and flour a 12-hole sponge finger mould. Spoon
the mixture into the moulds, then transfer the tin to the
oven and bake for 12 minutes.

Test with a wooden toothpick, if it comes out clean,
the cakes are done. Transfer the cakes to a wire rack
and leave to cool.

Amaretti Biscuits

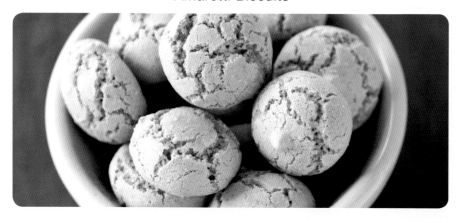

Makes 36
52 calories each
Prep time: 15 minutes
Cooking time: 15 minutes

2 large egg whites, 175 g ground almonds, 175 g
icing (confectioners') sugar, 1 tbsp amaretto liqueur

Preheat the oven to 160°C (140° fan) / 325F
/ gas 3 and oil a large baking tray.

Whisk the egg whites to stiff peaks in a
clean bowl then carefully fold in the almonds,
sugar and amaretto.

Spoon the mixture into a piping bag fitted
with a large plain nozzle and pipe 2 ½ cm /
1" rounds onto the baking tray.

Bake for 15 minutes or until golden brown
and crisp. Transfer to a wire rack to cool.

Bruschetta

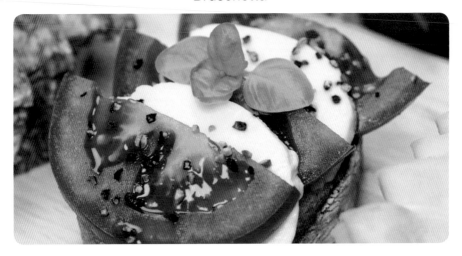

Serves 4
91 calories per serving
Prep time: 5 minutes
Cooking time: 2 minutes

4 slices of baguette
1 medium tomato
1 ball of light mozzarella
4 sprigs of basil

Toast the bread lightly in a toaster
or under a hot grill.

Cut the tomato in half, then cut each half into
6 slices. Cut the mozzarella into 8 slices.

Arrange alternate slices of tomato and mozzarella
on top of the baguette, then garnish with basil
and sprinkle with black pepper.

Blue Smoothie

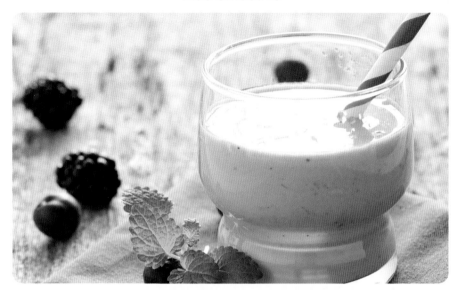

Serves 2
118 calories per serving
Prep time: **5 minutes**

50 g blueberries
50 g blackberries
100 g 0% fat Greek yoghurt
1 navel orange, juiced
1 tbsp runny honey

Put all of the
ingredients in a liquidiser
and blend until smooth.

Pour into two
glasses and serve.

Herb Straws

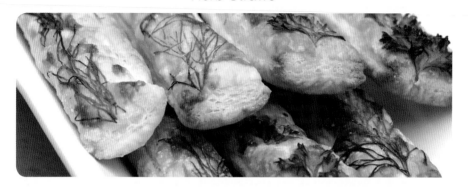

Makes 14
103 calories per serving
Prep time: **10 minutes**
Cooking time: **12 minutes**

320 g ready-rolled puff pastry
1 large egg, beaten
a small bunch of curly parsley
a small bunch of dill

Preheat the oven to 220°C (200° fan) / 425F / gas 7 and line a baking tray with greaseproof paper.

Cut the pastry across into 14 strips with the help of a ruler – each one should be 2.5 cm / 1 " wide. Brush the pastry strips with egg, then top 7 of them with parsley leaves and 7 with dill fronds.

Transfer the strips to the baking tray and bake for 12 minutes or until brown and crisp.

Watermelon Granita

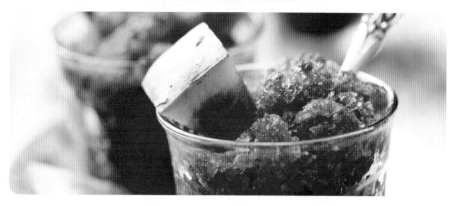

Serves 4
115 calories per serving
Prep time: **5 minutes**
Freezing time: **2 hours**

800 g watermelon,
peeled and deseeded
2 limes, juiced
50 g caster sugar

Cube the watermelon and put in
a blender with the lime juice and
caster sugar. Blend until smooth
then scrape the mixture into a
plastic tub and cover with a lid.

Freeze for 2 hours or until almost
firm then scrape the mixture into
icy grains with a fork.

Spoon into glasses and serve
immediately.

Exercise

Moving magic

Now's the time to get moving! The more active you are the better for your all-round health. Keeping physically busy can boost your metabolism. Being sedentary – sitting around for long periods – can lead to weight gain, especially around the middle. If you'd like a chance at that hourglass figure again, then jump up now and get going.

Many of us sit down at work, at a desk, or computer. Even more of us watch TV or read as a way of winding down. You don't need to give up your favourite pastimes, just break up periods of sitting with moving about.

Even if you only get up to make a cup of tea during your favourite programme, it can help. Perhaps walk while you're on the phone or use the stairs instead of an escalator or lift.

Why bother?

Keeping active every day helps keep your heart healthy, reduces your risk of serious illness and strengthens muscles and bones.

It can help give you better results while you're dieting too

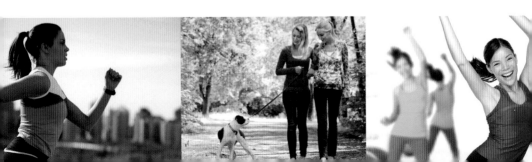

If you're new to exercise or have any underlying health conditions that might affect your ability to exercise safely, do consult your GP or medical practitioner before going ahead.

- helping your weight loss and toning up muscles as well.

You don't have to join a gym and pay expensive memberships to get fitter either. There are plenty of simple ways to build activity into your day.

It may seem hard to get started, especially if you've been leading a sedentary lifestyle for a while. But when you do, you'll feel a great sense of achievement - and you'll get a confidence boost too!

Don't sign up for a marathon if you struggle to walk to the post box. Start slowly and build up gradually. You'll be thrilled to see how quickly you feel the benefits. Check with your GP to make sure they're happy with your ideas for getting more active too.

Get going!

You don't have to set a whole hour aside every day to exercise. You get the best results if you fit exercise into your daily routine.

Start with something small and do it every day if you can. Before long, exercising will become second nature - and you're more likely to keep it up.

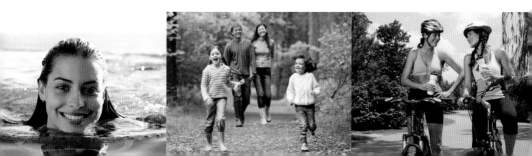

Walk this way

Go on, open your front door. Pop your shoes on and off you go. Get walking! It's a great way to boost morale, get fitter and tone up – and it's the cheapest exercise of all. No special equipment required, no hi-tech clothing, no groups to join. Just put one foot in front of the other and you're off.

Striding out

Start simply. If you have a dog, up your pace on their daily walks - or take them out more often. No dog ever says no to walkies! If you don't own a pet, ask a neighbour if you could take theirs for a trot round the block. Most dogs love an extra outing in the fresh air – they don't mind who takes them.

You don't even need a dog to make the most of walking. All you need is a comfortable pair of shoes and you're ready to go.

Wherever you live – in the city, town or country, there are masses of places to walk. And when you're on foot, you see the world differently – you notice more of your surroundings, from the birds in the trees, to the interesting buildings around you.

Make walking part of your everyday life and you'll be taking the first steps to a happier, healthier life. Try to make your walk active – as brisk as you feel comfortable with. That way you'll help burn calories quicker and get places faster!

Ring the changes on your walks.

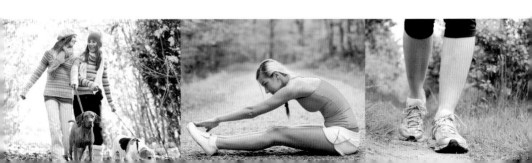

Why not:

- walk to the shops once a week to buy yourself a healthy treat.

- get your friends to come along. It can be a great way to catch up and exercise at the same time.

- vary your pace. That hill won't seem so steep once you've conquered it a few times!

- challenge yourself – start slowly and build up so that you can walk briskly for 10 then 20 then 30 minutes without getting out of breath. But remember, walking must be enjoyable to get the optimum benefits for you.

- change your routes. If you get bored with your local area, hop on a bus and seek out new haunts. Try a different park, a walk along the canal or stride out along rural footpaths.

- go a different way on different days – take a circular walk one day, then try an A-to-B route another day. Combine it with things you love – a walk to the cinema and back, a trip to the library, a walk to the railway station for a day out.

- enjoy the weather, rain or shine. Just make sure you're dressed for the climate. And if you go out walking when it's dark, stay safe by choosing well-lit areas with plenty of activity. Wear light or fluorescent clothing to make yourself more visible.

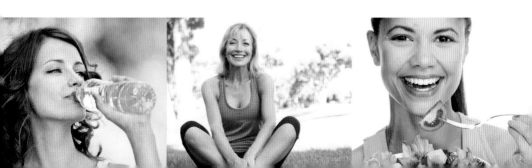

Stuck for ideas?

Get moving with these great ideas for improving your fitness.

Dance away

Get dancing! This can be anything from boogying round the kitchen to your favourite tunes or going to an organised class. Check out the local notice boards for details of groovy moving classes like zumba. You'll have so much fun it won't even feel like exercise!

Four minutes

That's the latest theory – that four minutes of intensive interval training is all you need to boost your fitness. Ask at your local gym. Or if that all seems a bit too good to be true join a standard interval training class. This involves doing short bursts (usually two minutes each) of exercise targeting specific areas of the body – from legs, to arms, to abs, giving you an all-round cardio workout that also tones vital muscle groups.

Swim

This is one of the cheapest forms of organised exercise and brilliant if you're new to the game. You can build up slowly and do a little bit more each time. Many local pools offer low-cost sessions. Swimming's easy to fit round your other commitments – go early in the morning to set yourself up for the day, or use it as a wind-down after work or when the day's chores are done.

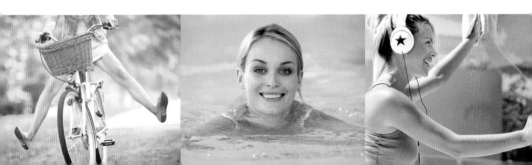

Clean it!

Use the smallest attachment when you vacuum the house and really put some effort in when you clean the windows. Working up a bit of a sweat means you'll burn more calories and your home will be sparkling to boot.

Car wash

Don't pay to go through a car wash. Clean it yourself with a bucket and sponge and plenty of elbow grease.

Get on your bike

If you have a bike, dust it off and get cycling. If you can cycle to work, try that. The fresh air will boost your mood and improve your sleep too.

Ditch the lift

If you normally take the lift, walk instead. Every little bit of extra exercise can help shed those pounds.

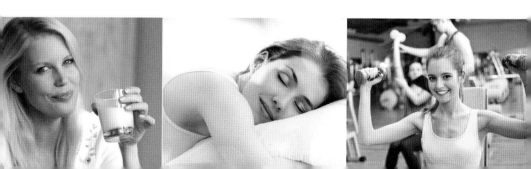

Week ① Measurements:

Bust   Waist   Hips

Today
I weigh:

Day 1   Total cals:

Breakfast:

Lunch:

Dinner:

Snacks:

Exercise:

Top tip
What's the small change you can make today and repeat tomorrow? Maybe you could fit in an extra 10 minutes of exercise or choose some new and exciting vegetables to rustle up a salad!

Day 2   Total cals:

Breakfast:

Lunch:

Dinner:

Snacks:

Exercise:

Day 3

Total cals:

Breakfast:

Lunch:

Dinner:

Snacks:

Exercise:

Day 4

Total cals:

Breakfast:

Lunch:

Dinner:

Snacks:

Exercise:

Day 5

Total cals:

Breakfast:

Lunch:

Dinner:

Snacks:

Exercise:

Day 6

Total cals:

Breakfast:

Lunch:

Dinner:

Snacks:

Exercise:

Did you know?

Dieting with a friend can help keep you on track.
Swap ideas and motivate each other to keep going.

Day 7

Total cals:

Breakfast:

Lunch:

Dinner:

Snacks:

Exercise:

Try this

Don't let yourself get too hungry. That's a sure fire way of ending
up with your hand in the biscuit tin. If a mealtime seems a long
way off, choose a snack to stave off the hunger pangs.

Week ②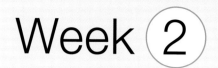

Today I weigh:

Weight loss so far:

Welcome to Week 2. This is the week that some people find hardest, so remember that and tell yourself you'll be fine. Just fine. After Week One you usually get quite a big weight loss as your body adjusts. From here on in, you'll possibly lose weight a little slower, but you WILL be losing.

Day 1

Total cals:

Breakfast:

Lunch:

Dinner:

Snacks:

Exercise:

Day 2

Total cals:

Breakfast:

Lunch:

Dinner:

Snacks:

Exercise:

Day 3

Total cals:

Breakfast:

Lunch:

Dinner:

Snacks:

Exercise:

Day 4

Total cals:

Breakfast:

Lunch:

Dinner:

Snacks:

Exercise:

Day 5

Total cals:

Breakfast:

Lunch:

Dinner:

Snacks:

Exercise:

Day 6

Total cals:

Breakfast:

Lunch:

Dinner:

Snacks:

Exercise:

Top tip

Boredom can lead to cheating. If you've been choosing the same breakfast every day so far, it's time to select one of the other early rising options.

Day 7

Total cals:

Breakfast:

Lunch:

Dinner:

Snacks:

Exercise:

Did you know?

Positive thinking works wonders! Tell yourself how well you're doing and give yourself a virtual pat on the back!

Week ③

You're working wonders! Those jeans feel looser already.
Enjoy every bite this week.

Day 1   Total cals:

Breakfast:

Lunch:

Dinner:

Snacks:

Exercise:

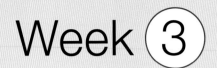

Top tip

Drink a glass of water with a slice of lemon and lime 15 minutes
before a meal. It cleanses your palate and helps you feel satisfied.

Day 2   Total cals:

Breakfast:

Lunch:

Dinner:

Snacks:

Exercise:

Day 3

Total cals:

Breakfast:

Lunch:

Dinner:

Snacks:

Exercise:

Day 4

Total cals:

Breakfast:

Lunch:

Dinner:

Snacks:

Exercise:

Day 5

Total cals:

Breakfast:

Lunch:

Dinner:

Snacks:

Exercise:

Day 6

Total cals:

Breakfast:

Lunch:

Dinner:

Snacks:

Exercise:

Did you know?

Berries are really low in calories and high in fibre and vitamin C. That goes for all berries – strawberries, raspberries and blackberries. So keep a punnet of them to hand to bulk up your snack options.

Day 7

Total cals:

Breakfast:

Lunch:

Dinner:

Snacks:

Exercise:

Try This

Get a couple of early nights every week. It works wonders for your moods and means you'll wake up feeling really refreshed. It stops you getting an attack of the late-night munchies too.

Week 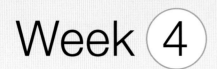4

Today I weigh:

Weight loss so far:

You're totally rocking! In Week 4, you'll probably find that you're really enjoying your food more than ever. Savour every mouthful on the road to the new you.

Day 1

Total cals:

Breakfast:

Lunch:

Dinner:

Snacks:

Exercise:

Day 2

Total cals:

Breakfast:

Lunch:

Dinner:

Snacks:

Exercise:

Day 3

Total cals:

Breakfast:

Lunch:

Dinner:

Snacks:

Exercise:

Day 4

Total cals:

Breakfast:

Lunch:

Dinner:

Snacks:

Exercise:

Day 5

Total cals:

Breakfast:

Lunch:

Dinner:

Snacks:

Exercise:

Day 6

Total cals:

Breakfast:

Lunch:

Dinner:

Snacks:

Exercise:

Top tip

Check out your bra! Dieting changes your body shape and after four weeks you might find that you need a tighter fastening or a new cup size.

Day 7

Total cals:

Breakfast:

Lunch:

Dinner:

Snacks:

Exercise:

Did you know?

Building up your exercise plan gradually can ensure that you stick to it and make it part of your life. Make sure you have lots of variety. Check out your local fitness centre. They do loads of fun classes – you're bound to find something you fancy.

Stage ① success!

Four whole weeks have passed and you're already looking much slimmer! There's a sparkle in your eyes and a spring in your step. Let's see how well you've done.

Step on the scales

Today I weigh

Weight loss to date

Take those measurements

Bust	Waist	Hips

You've stuck to the diet for four weeks now. That deserves a prize.

Here are a few ideas.

Active Reward

Treat yourself to a pedometer to check out how many steps you do every day. If you have a desk job, it's probably only around 3,000. Aim to take a few more steps every day until you reach 10,000.

Pamper Reward

Walk (yes, leave the car behind!) to the shops and treat yourself to your favourite magazine.

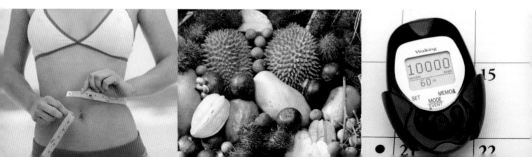

Then buy some sensationally scented bubble bath. Go home, close the bathroom door and sink into a frothy bath and read to your heart's content.

Yummy Reward

Next time you go food shopping choose yourself an exotic piece of fruit to spice up your dessert choices. How about a starfruit or a papaya? Maybe a juicy mango is your thing? Remember, most fruits are low in calories but high in vitamin C and they contain fibre to keep things moving.

Place a photo here of yourself, 4 weeks on.

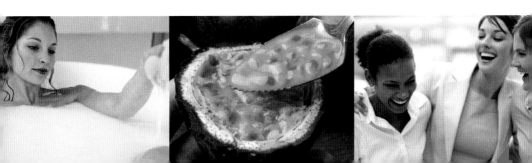

Week ⑤

Today I weigh:

Weight loss so far:

You're looking fab. People are commenting on it, aren't they? What's more, you can't keep that huge grin off your face. There's no stopping you now!

Day 1

Total cals:

Breakfast:

Lunch:

Dinner:

Snacks:

Exercise:

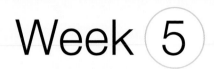

Top tip

Missing ice cream? Try a frozen yoghurt instead. Pop a pot in the freezer for half an hour then rip off the lid and tuck in. Try it!

Day 2

Total cals:

Breakfast:

Lunch:

Dinner:

Snacks:

Exercise:

Day 3

Total cals:

Breakfast:

Lunch:

Dinner:

Snacks:

Exercise:

Day 4

Total cals:

Breakfast:

Lunch:

Dinner:

Snacks:

Exercise:

Day 5

Total cals:

Breakfast:

Lunch:

Dinner:

Snacks:

Exercise:

Day 6

Total cals:

Breakfast:

Lunch:

Dinner:

Snacks:

Exercise:

Did you know?

Having a clear out can revive a flagging mood. If you find yourself feeling a bit down, clear out that kitchen cupboard or tackle your undies drawer. Getting neat and tidy is a real booster.

Day 7

Total cals:

Breakfast:

Lunch:

Dinner:

Snacks:

Exercise:

Try this

Treat yourself to a body exfoliating scrub and a bottle of body lotion. Next time you have a shower, massage your skin with the scrub, rinse and dry and apply a good dollop of body lotion. Slim and smooth...mmm!

Week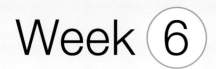

Today I weigh:

Weight loss so far:

You're at the half way mark now and the scales are already proof of your determination to stay on track. You're doing a brilliant job of eating a wide range of healthy foods and it shows!

Day 1

Total cals:

Breakfast:

Lunch:

Dinner:

Snacks:

Exercise:

Day 2

Total cals:

Breakfast:

Lunch:

Dinner:

Snacks:

Exercise:

Day 3

Total cals:

Breakfast:

Lunch:

Dinner:

Snacks:

Exercise:

Day 4

Total cals:

Breakfast:

Lunch:

Dinner:

Snacks:

Exercise:

Day 5

Total cals:

Breakfast:

Lunch:

Dinner:

Snacks:

Exercise:

Day 6

Total cals:

Breakfast:

Lunch:

Dinner:

Snacks:

Exercise:

Top tip

Had a bad day? Don't beat yourself up over it. Dieting can be like falling off a horse. You need to dust yourself off, give yourself a virtual hug and get straight back on track.

Day 7

Total cals:

Breakfast:

Lunch:

Dinner:

Snacks:

Exercise:

Try this

Try not to do anything else while eating. Don't work on the computer or eat while walking along. It's easy to eat more if you're distracted. Concentrate on your food and enjoy every mouthful.

Week ⑦

Today I weigh:

Weight loss so far:

Not long to go now and those clothes look looser. Well done! Keep smiling and keep going! Why not up your exercise this week to really see results?

Day 1

Total cals:

Breakfast:

Lunch:

Dinner:

Snacks:

Exercise:

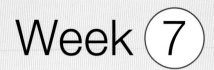

Top tip

Keep recording your eating habits. Remember to write down everything – even if you have a bad day.

Day 2

Total cals:

Breakfast:

Lunch:

Dinner:

Snacks:

Exercise:

Day 3

Total cals:

Breakfast:

Lunch:

Dinner:

Snacks:

Exercise:

Day 4

Total cals:

Breakfast:

Lunch:

Dinner:

Snacks:

Exercise:

Day 5

Total cals:

Breakfast:

Lunch:

Dinner:

Snacks:

Exercise:

Day 6

Total cals:

Breakfast:

Lunch:

Dinner:

Snacks:

Exercise:

Did you know?

Visualising yourself slim can help you keep on track.
Close your eyes and imagine how great it will feel to fit
into those jeans again.

Day 7

Total cals:

Breakfast:

Lunch:

Dinner:

Snacks:

Exercise:

Try this

Know your danger times. If you often get the munchies after
dinner, make sure you have a healthy snack ready so you're
not tempted to nip out for a takeaway.

Week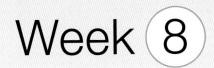

Today I weigh:

Weight loss so far:

Two thirds of the diet plan is behind you now. It'll all be plain sailing so long as you don't get over-confident and start cutting corners. Your dream body is well within reach!

Day 1
Total cals:

Breakfast:

Lunch:

Dinner:

Snacks:

Exercise:

Day 2
Total cals:

Breakfast:

Lunch:

Dinner:

Snacks:

Exercise:

Day 3

Total cals:

Breakfast:

Lunch:

Dinner:

Snacks:

Exercise:

Day 4

Total cals:

Breakfast:

Lunch:

Dinner:

Snacks:

Exercise:

Day 5

Total cals:

Breakfast:

Lunch:

Dinner:

Snacks:

Exercise:

Day 6

Total cals:

Breakfast:

Lunch:

Dinner:

Snacks:

Exercise:

Top tip

Don't eat in front of the TV. It's easy to put more in your mouth when you're concentrating on your favourite soap. Instead, sit at the table in another room and only turn on the telly when you've finished.

Day 7

Total cals:

Breakfast:

Lunch:

Dinner:

Snacks:

Exercise:

Did you know?

Don't be tempted to step on the scales more than once a week. If the scales don't show the results you're expecting then it can leave you fed up and tempted to munch on high calorie snacks. If they show better results, it can tempt you to slacken off!

Stage ② success!

Eight weeks in! Look how far you've come and how well you're doing. Just set your sights on your final goal and you'll be a winner.

Step on the scales

Today I weigh	
Weight loss to date	

Take those measurements

Bust	Waist	Hips

Active Reward

If you've been striding out getting those steps in, then now's the time to treat yourself to some sports gear. It doesn't need to cost the earth. If your budget's tight, choose a pair of new sports' socks. If you're feeling flush, splash out on a new pair of trainers to put an extra spring in your step.

Pamper Reward

You're looking slimmer already and your hair is gorgeous and glossy. Maybe it's time for a new style or colour. Chat to your hairdresser and book an

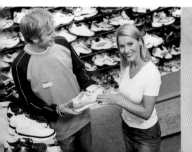
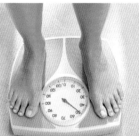
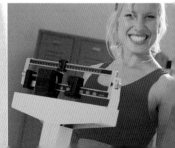

appointment so that your hair truly is the crowning glory of your dieting days. A new hairdo is always a cracking confidence boost.

Yummy Reward

If you've been sticking to boring old cucumber, lettuce and tomato for your salad requirements then branch out and get colourful. Make your salads sing on your plate with the addition of bright coloured vegetables. Remember, we eat with our eyes first, so add red and yellow peppers, maybe some colourful shredded red

cabbage and purple beetroot for a real rainbow on your plate!

Place a
photo here
of yourself,
8 weeks on.

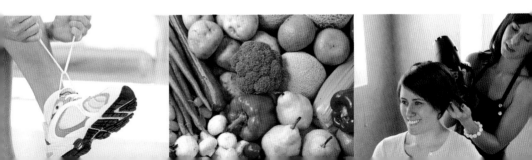

Week 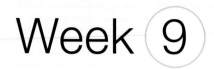 9

Today I weigh:

Weight loss so far:

Woo-hoo! You're an old hand at this dieting lark now. And look how different you feel than you did in the beginning. Your confidence is glowing!

Day 1   Total cals:

Breakfast:

Lunch:

Dinner:

Snacks:

Exercise:

Top tip
If someone offers you a biscuit just say, no thanks, I've just eaten. That way you don't offend anyone but don't wreck your progress either!

Day 2   Total cals:

Breakfast:

Lunch:

Dinner:

Snacks:

Exercise:

Day 3

Total cals:

Breakfast:

Lunch:

Dinner:

Snacks:

Exercise:

Day 4

Total cals:

Breakfast:

Lunch:

Dinner:

Snacks:

Exercise:

Day 5

Total cals:

Breakfast:

Lunch:

Dinner:

Snacks:

Exercise:

Day 6

Total cals:

Breakfast:

Lunch:

Dinner:

Snacks:

Exercise:

Did you know?

You can control comfort eating! If you've had a bad day don't be tempted to pig out. Take some deep breaths and close your eyes for a few moments. You'll be surprised how quickly the urge to binge passes.

Day 7

Total cals:

Breakfast:

Lunch:

Dinner:

Snacks:

Exercise:

Try this

Use your friends! Ask them to keep naughty chocolate and cakes away from you as you near your goal. Maybe even encourage them to join you if you know they want to shed a few pounds.

Week 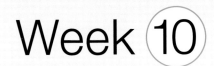 10

Today I weigh:

Weight loss so far:

Yikes! You really are a super slimming whiz-kid. And you're desperate to buy new clothes too. Hang on until week 12 though or you might have to go shopping all over again!

Day 1

Total cals:

Breakfast:

Lunch:

Dinner:

Snacks:

Exercise:

Day 2

Total cals:

Breakfast:

Lunch:

Dinner:

Snacks:

Exercise:

Day 3

Total cals:

Breakfast:

Lunch:

Dinner:

Snacks:

Exercise:

Day 4

Total cals:

Breakfast:

Lunch:

Dinner:

Snacks:

Exercise:

Day 5

Total cals:

Breakfast:

Lunch:

Dinner:

Snacks:

Exercise:

Day 6

Total cals:

Breakfast:

Lunch:

Dinner:

Snacks:

Exercise:

Top tip

Make a rewards jar of all the things you enjoy. Think of things that appeal to your senses, sight, sound, touch etc – like watching the sunset, lying in the sun for an hour, reading a book. Jot them on pieces of paper and pop in a jar. Pull one out at random when you feel you deserve it.

Day 7

Total cals:

Breakfast:

Lunch:

Dinner:

Snacks:

Exercise:

Try this

Really enjoy your favourite foods - if you tell yourself everything is banned, you'll crave it more.

Week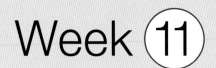

Today I weigh:

Weight loss so far:

The end is in sight and your energy is shining. If you have a partner or kids, they're thrilled with the new you. But this is your journey, so don't give up yet!

Day 1   Total cals:

Breakfast:

Lunch:

Dinner:

Snacks:

Exercise:

Top tip

Enjoy your treats away from home. For example if you love a frothy coffee, walk to your local coffee shop and burn calories on the way!

Day 2   Total cals:

Breakfast:

Lunch:

Dinner:

Snacks:

Exercise:

Day 3

Total cals:

Breakfast:

Lunch:

Dinner:

Snacks:

Exercise:

Day 4

Total cals:

Breakfast:

Lunch:

Dinner:

Snacks:

Exercise:

Day 5

Total cals:

Breakfast:

Lunch:

Dinner:

Snacks:

Exercise:

Day 6

Total cals:

Breakfast:

Lunch:

Dinner:

Snacks:

Exercise:

Did you know?

People who lose weight steadily and sensibly are more likely to keep it off unlike people who crash diet.

Day 7

Total cals:

Breakfast:

Lunch:

Dinner:

Snacks:

Exercise:

Try this

Eating out? Order children's portions or choose a side dish as a main meal. You may get some quizzical looks but most restaurants are happy to help.

Week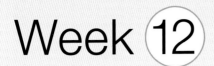

One week to go... It's the final push so make sure you stay right on track this week. It's the last week so make it your best so far. Concentrate on choosing your favourites from the meal suggestions and dream on for the new you!

Day 1
Total cals:

Breakfast:

Lunch:

Dinner:

Snacks:

Exercise:

Day 2
Total cals:

Breakfast:

Lunch:

Dinner:

Snacks:

Exercise:

Day 3

Total cals:

Breakfast:

Lunch:

Dinner:

Snacks:

Exercise:

Day 4

Total cals:

Breakfast:

Lunch:

Dinner:

Snacks:

Exercise:

Day 5

Total cals:

Breakfast:

Lunch:

Dinner:

Snacks:

Exercise:

Day 6

Total cals:

Breakfast:

Lunch:

Dinner:

Snacks:

Exercise:

Top tip

Plan for the occasional slice of cheesecake. If you know it's coming, you'll be better prepared. Cut back a little bit at first, then you won't feel guilty.

Day 7

Total cals:

Breakfast:

Lunch:

Dinner:

Snacks:

Exercise:

Did you know?

Keep drinking plenty of water and low calorie drinks.
We often think we're hungry when in fact we're just thirsty.

Stage ③ success!

Yay!! You've done it! You've stuck to the plan for 12 whole weeks and now you're lighter and probably feeling full of energy.

If you've been following the plan, chances are your skin will be looking lovely thanks to all the fruit and vegetables you've been munching on.

The moment of truth

Step on the scales then and believe in yourself. Close your eyes. Open them again. Yes! You're a weight loss wonder.

Today I weigh

In 12 weeks I've lost an amazing

I measure...

Bust	Waist	Hips

Active Reward

If you've been swimming to keep fit, splash out on a new cossie, one that shows off your slim and toned new curves.

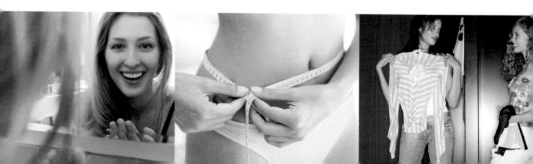

Or if you've been doing lots of dog walking, treat your pooch to a new collar and lead. That way, every time you go walkies, it will be a reminder of how well you've done.

Pamper Reward

You've been waiting to do this, be honest. Clothes shopping! Even if it's just a new top or a drawerful of undies, go for it. But don't splurge too fast. Work out what you really want and be prepared to try things on. Chances are, you'll be selecting a smaller size too!

Place a photo here of yourself, 12 weeks on.

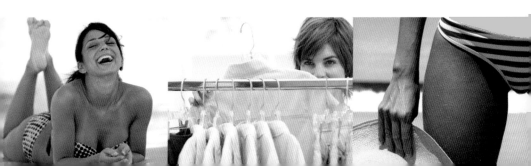

Calories List

All calorie counts are approximate and intended as a guide only. For branded foods, check the packaging where all calorie and fat contents are usually displayed.

Dairy Products

Butter, 10g	75
Cheese, Edam, 40g	135
Cheese, Feta, 40g	100
Cheese, Cheddar, 40g	165
Cottage cheese, 50g	50
Cream, clotted, 1 tablespoon	175
Cream, double, 1 tablespoon	45
Egg, large, single	90
Egg, medium, single	80
Milk, whole, 250ml/half pt	175
Milk, semi skimmed, 250ml/half pt	125
Milk, skimmed, 250ml/half pt	95
Sunflower spread, 10g	65
Sunflower spread, light, 10g	28

Yoghurt, natural, 150g pot	130
Yoghurt, fruit, low fat, 150g pot	110
Yoghurt, fruit, fat-free, 125g pot	60

Breads and Cereals

Bagel, plain, 85g	235
Branflakes, 30g	120
Bread, white, 1 40g slice	100
Bread, wholemeal, 40g slice	90
Brioche roll, 35g	130
Burger bun, 85g	225
Cornflakes, 30g	120
Crispbread, Ryvita, 4 slices	120
Croissant, 40g	185
Crumpet, 40g	80
Naan bread, 160g	455
Panini, 85g	235
Porridge Oats, 50g	180
Tortilla, plain, 55g	150
Weetabix, 2 biscuits	135

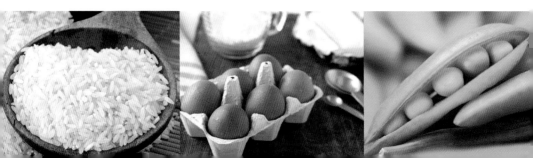

Cakes and Pastries

Apple turnover, average 1	315
Battenberg cake, average 40g	150
Chocolate mini rolls, average	125
Chocolate muffin, average 75g	320
Chocolate Swiss roll, average slice, 25g	100
Croissant, average 45g	185
Crumpets, average 1	100
Doughnut, jam, average 75g	250
English muffins, white, 1	160
English muffins, wholemeal, 1	155
Hot cross bun, 70g, each	220
Lemon and poppyseed muffin, average 90g	380
Mince Pie, average 55g	240
Pain au Chocolat, average 60g	240
Pain au Raisin, average	345
Scone, fruit, average 70g	255
Swiss roll, 30g slice	85

Chocolate and Nibbles

Chocolate, milk, 100g	500
Chocolate, dark, 100g	500
Chocolate, white, 100g	535
Crisps, 25g	135
Peanuts, salted, 25g	150
Cashew nuts, 25g	155
Popcorn, salted, 44g	240
Popcorn, sweet, 44g	290

Top tip

Trim meat of all
visible fat and remove the
skin from poultry. When buying
minced meat, opt for the
extra lean pack.

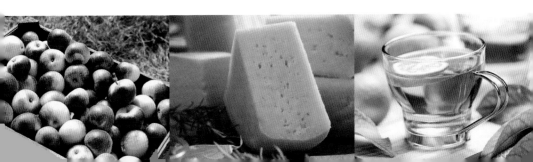

Biscuits

Bourbon Creams, 2 average	140
Chocolate chip cookies, 2 average	100
Custard Creams, 2	130
Digestives, chocolate, 2	180
Digestives, plain, 2 average	160
Fig rolls, 2 average	140
Garibaldi, 2 average	80
Ginger nuts, 2 average	90
Rich Tea, 2 average	80
Shortbread fingers, 1	100

Pasta and Rice

Pasta, wholemeal penne, 75g	240
Pasta, wholemeal spaghetti, 75g	245
Pasta, white penne, 75g	270
Pasta, white spaghetti, 75g	265
Rice, brown, 75g	265
Rice, basmati white, 75g	270
Rice, Arborio risotto, 75g	265

Meat, fish and poultry

Bacon, two lean rashers, 42g	100
Beef mince, 21% fat, 125g	230
Chicken breast, skinless average	170
Cod, fillet, 140g	115
Haddock, grilled, 120g	125
Ham, 25g	30
Herring, grilled, 110g	200
Lamb, lean diced, 125g	220
Mussels, weighed with shells, 90g	25
Plaice, grilled, 130g	125
Prawns, peeled, 110g	90
Salmon fillet, 115g	245
Sausages, pork, 100g (2)	260
Sirloin steak, grilled, 175g	375
Squid, 140g	115
Stewing steak, lean, 140g	260
Tuna, in brine, 100g drained	105
Tuna, in oil, 100g drained	190
Turkey breast, 100g	100

Top tip

Choose high fibre options
- go for wholemeal bread
instead of white and choose
wholegrain cereals
and pasta too.

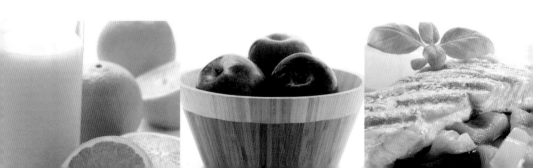

Fruit, fresh

Apple, eating, 100g	50
Banana, medium 165g	100
Cherries, 100g	50
Figs, average 55g	25
Gooseberries, 80g	35
Grapes, seedless, 100g	70
Grapefruit, average	35
Guava, average	40
Kiwi fruit, average	40
Lychees, 100g	65
Mango, 100g	60
Melon, cantaloupe, 150g	30
Melon, galia, 150g	35
Melon, honeydew, 150g	40
Nectarine, average	60
Orange, large	80
Papaya, average	50
Passion fruit, average	15
Pear, average	60
Peaches, average	35
Pineapple, fresh, 100g	45
Plum, average	20
Pomegranate, average	50
Raspberries, 100g	30
Rhubarb, 100g	10
Satsumas, average	50
Strawberries, 100g	30
Watermelon, 200g	70

Top tip

Use a smaller plate
to make your portions
look more filling.

Fruit, dried

Apricots, 100g	160
Banana chips, 100g	540
Currants, 100g	170
Dates, 100g	270
Figs, 100g	225
Prunes, 100g	140
Raisins, 100g	270
Sultanas, 100g	275

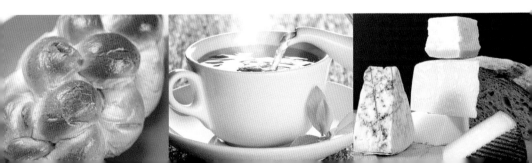

Spreads

Cheese triangle, average	45
Chocolate/hazelnut spread, 1 tablespoon	85
Fish paste, 2 teaspoons	20
Honey, 1 tablespoon	60
Jam, fruit, 1 tablespoon	40
Lemon curd, 1 tablespoon	40
Marmalade, 1 tablespoon	40
Marmite (yeast extract), 1teaspoon	10
Peanut butter, smooth or crunchy, 1 tablespoon	120

Vegetables

Asparagus, 80g	20
Aubergine, 80g	15
Beansprouts, 80g	25
Broccoli, 100g	40
Brussels sprouts, 80g	35
Cabbage,100g	30
Carrots, 100g	40
Cauliflower, 100g	40
Celery, 100g	10
Courgettes, 100g	10
Cucumber, 100g	10
Green beans, 100g	25
Leeks, 100g	20
Lettuce, 100g	15
Mushrooms, 100g	15
Onions, 100g	35
Parsnips, 100g	75
Peas, 100g	70
Peppers, 100g green or red	15
Potatoes, 250g	200
Rocket, 100g	20
Spinach, fresh, 100g	25
Squash, butternut, 80g	30
Swede, flesh only, 100g	10
Sweet Potatoes, 100g	95
Tomatoes, fresh, 1	15
Watercress, 100g	20

Sauces and Dressings

Brown sauce, 1 tablespoon	20
French dressing, 1 tablespoon	95
Horseradish sauce, 1 tablespoon	30
Mayonnaise, 1 tablespoon	200
Mayonnaise, light, 1 tablespoon	85
Mustard, 1 teaspoon	10
Salad Cream, 1 tablespoon	70
Soy Sauce, 1 tablespoon	10
Tomato ketchup, 1 tablespoon	25

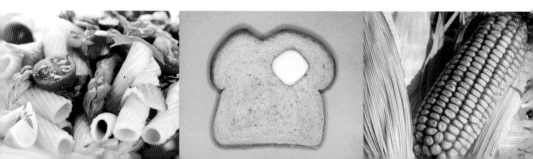

Canned Foods

Baked beans, in tomato sauce, 210g	185
Black eyed beans, 125g	145
Butter beans, 120g	125
Chickpeas, 200g	200
Corned beef, 100g	225
Kidney beans, 120g	125
Peas, processed, 90g	90
Spaghetti hoops, in tomato sauce, 205g	115
Sweetcorn, 80g	55

Soft Drinks

Apple juice, 200ml	75
Cola, 330ml can	135
Ginger Ale, 150ml	30
Lemonade, 300ml can	75
Orange juice, 200ml	75
Pineapple juice, 200ml	85
Tomato juice, 200ml	30
Tonic Water, 150ml	50

Alcoholic Drinks

Alcoholic drinks vary in calorie content depending on the alcohol contained in them so be careful! It's easy to take in more calories than you think.

Beer, bitter, half pint/250ml	100
Cider, dry, 250ml	100
Cider, sweet, 250 ml	125
Lager, 250 ml, average	100
Spirits, 50ml, average	100
Wine, red dry, 100ml	70
Wine, rose, 100ml	70
Wine, sparkling white, 125ml	95
Wine, white dry, 125ml	100

Top tip

Choose skimmed or semi-skimmed milk and use reduce fat spreads.

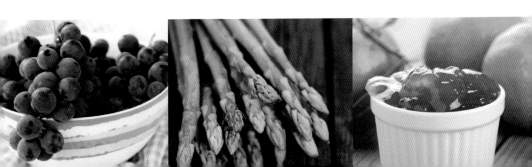

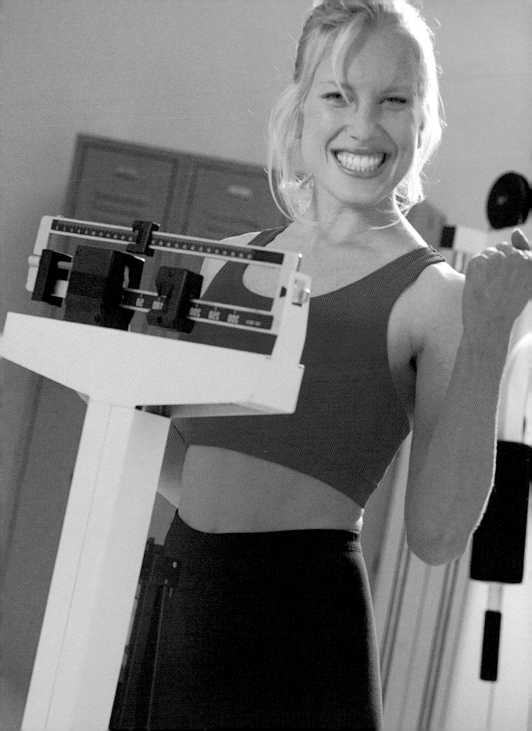